Directory for Medicinal Plants Conservation

Networks, Organizations, Projects, Information Sources

by Max Kasparek, Andreas Gröger and Uwe Schippmann

IUCN/SSC Medicinal Plant Specialist Group
German Federal Agency for Nature Conservation

Cover Picture: Market situation in Ozumba, Mexiko, D.F. (Uwe Schippmann, BfN)

IUCN/SSC Medicinal Plant Specialist Group

The *Species Survival Commission* (SSC) is one of the largest and most active of IUCN – *The World Conservation Union's* six volunteer commissions. The SSC network encompasses 7000 volunteer member scientists, field researchers, government officials and conservation leaders from 169 countries. Commission members, in addition to providing leadership for conservation efforts for specific animal and plant groups, contribute technical and scientific counsel to biodiversity conservation projects throughout the world. Commission members also serve as resources to governments, international conventions, and conservation organizations.

The SSC works primarily through its 110 Specialist Groups. The *Medicinal Plant Specialist Group* (MPSG) was established upon recommendation of the *Plant Conservation Subcommittee* in 1994 and comprises currently approximately 50 members. The Medicinal Plant Specialist Group is co-chaired by Dr A. B. Cunningham and Dr U. Schippmann.

German Federal Agency for Nature Conservation

The Federal Agency for Nature Conservation (Bundesamt für Naturschutz, BfN) is Germany's central federal scientific agency for national and international nature conservation and landscape management. Together with Federal Environment Agency and the Federal Agency for Radiation Protection, it is part of the Federal Ministry for the Environment's area of responsibility. The Federal Agency for Nature Conservation is located in Bonn. It maintains branch offices in Leipzig and on Vilm Island, near Rügen.

The Federal Agency for Nature Conservation conducts its own research and commissions outside research, advises the Federal Ministry for the Environment in the areas of national and international nature conservation, and supports major nature conservation projects, on the Länder level, as well as pilot projects relevant to nature conservation. It is responsible for permits for import and export of protected plant and animal species, and informs interested citizens about nature conservation.

Preparation: This directory has been prepared by Dr Max Kasparek, Bleichstr. 1,
69120 Heidelberg, Germany. Tel.: (+49) 6221/475069, Fax: (+49) 6221/471858,
e-mail: Kasparek@t-online.de.

Printed by LV Druck/Landwirtschaftsverlag GmbH, Münster

Orders: Copies of this directory can be ordered at a price of DM 19,80 from:
Landwirtschaftsverlag, Postfach 480249, D-48079 Münster
Tel.: (+49) 2501/801-117, Fax: (+49) 2501/801-204

ISBN 3-89624-606-2

Printed on acid-free paper

Preface

One of the main outcomes of the UN *Conference on Environment and Development*, Rio de Janeiro 1992, was the *Convention on Biological Diversity*. The main focus of this new Convention lies on the sustainable use of biological resources, resulting from the growing awareness of economic benefits inherent in biological diversity. This international framework tries to harmonize commercial interests with nature conservation necessities.

It is obvious that the implementation of the Biodiversity Convention is an extremely complex procedure. The effectiveness of sustainable use essentially depends on up-to-date information on the fragility or stability of the biological resource. This information must be made available to all parties using and managing the resource. In most cases, correspondent mechanisms for distributing the information do not exist.

In response to this need and recognising the importance and the limitation of medicinal plant resources, the Species Survival Commission of IUCN-The World Conservation Union, together with the Federal Agency for Nature Conservation of Germany, offer the *Directory for Medicinal Plants Conservation*. We hope this publication will assist the flow of information between policy makers, scientists and technical experts in the management of medicinal plant resources.

The Species Survival Commission leverages a small operating budget through the invaluable contributions of time and expertise its member scientists make and in-kind support provided by a wide variety of institutions, such as the Federal Agency for Nature Conservation of Germany. The *Directory for Medicinal Plants Conservation* demonstrates the conservation potential and value of these important partnerships.

Dr. George Rabb
Chairman
Species Survival Commission
IUCN-The World Conservation Union

Prof. Dr. Martin Uppenbrink
President
Federal Agency for Nature Conservation
Germany

Contents

Introduction

As many as 80% of the world's peoples depend on traditional medicine for their primary health care needs. The greater part of traditional therapy involves the use of medicinal plants or their extracts and active compounds. It is not just in developing countries that phytopharmaceuticals are widely used; the use of plant-based pharmaceuticals is making a come-back in developed countries as well.

The increased use of medicinal plants often leads to an over-exploitation of local populations. Many species are threatened. In a joint venture, the World Health Organization (WHO), IUCN–The World Conservation Union, and World Wide Fund for Nature (WWF) convened an International Consultation on the Conservation of Medicinal Plants, bringing together experts in various fields to exchange views and making recommendations for action. The consultation took place in March 1988 in Thailand. Subsequently *Guidelines on the Conservation of Medicinal Plants* were prepared which were published in 1993. Finally, the *IUCN / SSC Medicinal Plant Specialist Group* was founded in 1994 to take up the initiative, and this *Directory on Medicinal Plants Conservation* is a direct result of these efforts.

Medicinal plants play an increasing role in nature conservation. Whereas forests have for long been regarded more or less exclusively as a source for timber extraction, the value of their by-products, the „non-wood forest products", has only recently been fully understood. Medicinal plants are important non-wood forest products and they help to preserve the world's forests.

Many groups, organizations, institutions, and projects deal with medicinal plants. In this study, a first attempt has been made to compile information on these groups. Emphasis has been given to those which deal with conservation issues, but research and management have also been covered. The objective is to improve communication among those who are active in this field, to promulgate details on current initiatives, and to support the coordination of activities dealing with the same topic.

For the preparation of this directory, a questionnaire was sent out to groups already known to us from literature surveys and from previous personal contacts. In our questionnaire, we asked for information on the group and for recommendations concerning other groups and projects that we could contact. This kind of survey made it possible to obtain almost exclusively „recommended contacts".

Biodiversity prospecting and its policy implications for medicinal plants are recognized as an important issue in medicinal plants conservation. This directory, however, is focussing less on this than on other aspects of medicinal plants conservation. For those that want to follow up the role of medicinal plants in biodiversity prospecting, a few references are given below which are recommended for further reading.

All questionnaires returned to us by 31th May 1996 were used. Although an impressive number of groups sent us information on their organization and their work, we are fully aware that there are still many groups which were either not identified by us or which did not respond to our enquiry. We hope to have a more comprehensive coverage in a second edition of the directory which is tentatively scheduled for 1997. Additions, updates and corrections are also most welcome from the groups already covered now.

We hope that the users of the directory will benefit from it, and that the groups listed here will themselves be able to make new contacts for the benefit of their work.

Recommendations for further reading on biodiversity prospecting

Baker, J. T., R. P. Borris, B. Carte, G. A. Cordell, D. D. Soejarto, G. M. Cragg, M. P. Gupta, M. M. Iwu, D. R. Madulid & V. R. Tyler (1995): Natural pruduct drug discovery and development: new perspectives on international collaboration. – Journal of Natural Products 58: 1325–1357.

Cunningham, A. B. (1993): Ethics, ethnobiological research and biodiversity. – Report to World Wide Fund for Nature (WWF International).

King, S. R., T. J. Carlson & K. Moran (1996): Biological diversity, indigenous knowledge, drug discovery and intellectual property rights: creating reciprocity and maintaining relationship. – Journal of Ethnopharmacology 51: 45–57.

Laird, S. (1995): Fair deals in the search for new products. – Report to World Wide Fund for Nature (WWF International).

Reid, W. V., S. A. Laird, C. A. Meyer, R. Gamez, A. Sittenfeld, D. H. Janzen, M. A. Gollin & C. Juma (1993): Biodiversity prospecting. – World Resources Institute, Washington.

International Organizations

Global

Biodiversity Action Network (BIONET)

Status: Non-governmental organization with a total of approximately 230 members. BIONET was founded by US NGOs (esp. Conservation International, Defender of Wildlife, Environmental and Energy Study Institute, Sierra Club, and World Resources Institute) in 1993. BIONET members include nearly all the major US environmental groups and many other smaller organizations. Strictly speaking, BIONET is composed solely of U.S. NGOs, but the long-term goal is to expand the concept globally.

Objective:

- to strengthen biodiversity policy and law, most specifically for the effective implementation of the *Convention on Biological Diversity.*

Activities: BIONET provides a documentation service containing information related to the policy aspects of the usage of medicinal plants.

Geographic interest: World-wide.

Database: Membership directory.

Information/resources: A quarterly newsletter *Biodiversity Bulletin*, frequent reports, and updates on issues on the *Convention of Biological Diversity*.

Funding: Membership fees and donations by member organizations.

Contact person: Sheldon Cohen (coordinator).

Address: Biodiversity Action Network (BIONET), 1400 16th Street, N.W. Suite 502, Washington, D.C. 20036 U.S.A. Tel.: (+1) 202 / 547.8902, Fax: (+1) 202 / 265.0222, e-mail: bionet@igc.apc.org.

Global

Botanic Gardens Conservation International

Status: Botanic Gardens Conservation International (BGCI) is a non-governmental organization with a regular membership of approx. 500 in some 80 countries. It was founded in 1987 on the initiative of IUCN, the World Conservation Union.

Objectives:

- to link botanic gardens and arboreta as a co-operating global network for effective plant conservation.

Activities: The technical guidance, data and support for botanical gardens to further conservation techniques, to monitor illegal rare plant trade, and to assist in the reintroduction of cultivated plants to the wild, including medicinal plants.

Geographic interest: World-wide.

Database: A computer database has been developed on the rare plants in over 300 institutions, to bring worldwide co-ordination to the individual efforts of each garden.

Information/resources: The *Botanic Gardens Conservation News* and the *Roots Education Newsletter* are published bi-annually. In addition, a series of technical publications on a variety of subjects relating to botanic gardens and plant conservation is published. The *International Botanic Gardens Conservation Congress* is organized, and occasionally training courses on special topics are offered.

Funding: Funds are available through subscriptions, grants, donations and contracts.

Contact person: Dr. P. Wyse Jackson (Secretary-General).

Address: Botanic Gardens Conservation International, Descanso House, 199 Kew Road, Richmond, Surrey TW9 3BW, United Kingdom. Tel. (+44) 181 / 332-5953 (-5954, -5955), Fax (+44) 181 / 332-5956, e-mail: pwj@bgci.rbgkew.org.uk.

Centre for Economic Botany at the Royal Botanic Gardens Kew

Global

Status: The Royal Botanic Gardens, founded in the 18th century, is a non-departmental public body under the Ministry of Agriculture, Fisheries and Food of the United Kingdom.

Objectives:

- to foster better management of the earth's environment by increasing knowledge and understanding of the plant kingdom, the basis of life on earth.

Activities: The activities of the Royal Botanic Gardens at Kew cover a wide area in the fields of plant and fungal taxonomy, achieved through systematic, anatomical, morphological, biochemical, molecular etc. studies. It also has living collections representing in total 38,000 taxa. Specific activities on medicinal plants cover ethnobotany, with projects on anti-malaria research in Amazonia and wound-healing in the U.K., backed by extensive bioassaying for biological activity from plants worldwide. The Centre for Economic Botany is a partner in the *People and Plants Initiative* together with WWF and UNESCO.

Geographic interest: World-wide.

Database: There are several computerized databases on different aspects of botany. None of them is specific for medicinal plants, but most of them contain information on medicinal plants.

Information/resources: The *Kew Bulletin* is published four times per year. There are numerous bulletins, newsletters, meetings, congresses, workshops and seminars on specific topics.

Funding: 75% of the funds are made available through the British Government. The remaining 25% come from a variety of sources including visitor fees.

Contact person: Dr. Hew Prendergast.

Address: Centre for Economic Botany, Royal Botanic Gardens, Kew, Richmond, Surrey TW9 3AE, United Kingdom. Tel. (+44) 181 / 332-5206, Fax (+44) 181 / 332-5228.

Global

Chemical Industries Branch of UNIDO

Status: The *Chemical Industries Branch* is part of UNIDO, the *United Nations Industrial Development Organization*. It is a United Nations Agency.

Objectives:

- to develop the industrial utilization of medicinal and aromatic plants in developing countries
- to introduce systematic cultivation to minimize the effect on natural flora exploitation
- to introduce proper sustainable and protective harvesting methods, when harvesting from the wild is feasible
- to provide technical assistance in the fields of domestication, development of propagation material, post-harvest technology, processing, quality control and marketing
- to conserve biodiversity and to combat deforestation.

Activities: Current activities include ethnobotanical surveys and economic mapping of medicinal and aromatic plants, domestication, conservation through the introduction of systematic cultivation mostly of exploited natural flora. Industrial processing of non-wood forest products includes medicinal and aromatic plants. Formulation into pharmaceutical dosage forms and fragrances. In addition to medicinal plants, projects include plants used in cosmetics, gums, resins, colourants etc.

Geographic interest: Developing countries in Asia, Africa, Latin America and Eastern Europe.

Database: None.

Information/resources: Technical reports of consultants and irregular seminars and workshops.

Funding: Donor funds by member states of the United Nations. UNIDO has a funding capacity for projects on a cost-sharing basis. Collaborative projects are welcome.

Contact person: Prof. Dr. T. De Silva.

Address: Chemical Industries Branch, Industrial Sectors and Environment Division, United Nations Industrial Development Organization (UNIDO), P.O. Box 300, Vienna International Centre, 1400 Vienna, Austria. Tel. (+43) 1 / 21131-6819, Fax (+43) 1 / 21131-3946, e-mail: tde-silva@unido.org.

The Healing Forest Conservancy

Global

Status: Non-governmental organization with approximately 50 members. It was founded in 1990 by Shaman Pharmaceuticals Inc.

Objective:
- to develop and implement a process to compensate indigenous peoples and biodiversity-rich countries for the commercial use of their traditional knowledge of the use of medicinal plants for drug discovery.

Activities: After consulting with indigenous groups, the conservancy develops and holds pilot projects to test compensation options. Pilot projects are to demarcate a plant reserve for a healer association, and two brief programmes in India and Cameroun to train indigenous women (not excluding men) in ethnobotany basics and issues.

Geographic interest: Global.

Database: None.

Information/resources: Many publications in various journals, and regular seminars and meetings. Training courses in ethnobotany in India 1994 and in Cameroun in 1995.

Funding: Funds for the projects are received from industry, foundations, environmental NGOs, and the Government of the United

States. There is a funding capacity for projects of other groups and initiatives.

Contact person: Mrs. Kary Moran (executive director).

Address: The Healing Forest Conservancy, 3521 S Street, N.W., Washington, D.C. 20007, U.S.A. Tel./Fax: (+1) 202 / 333-3438.

Global

IDRC International Medicinal Plants Network

Status: The *International Medicinal Plants Network* is a research and development agency (donor) and is part of the Canadian *International Development Research Centre* (IDRC). It was founded in 1993 on the initiative of Dr. Cherla B. Sastry, who is still the director.

Objectives:
- to conserve biodiversity
- to generate enterprise
- to promote traditional medicine.

Activities: The *International Medicinal Plants Network* sponsors a wide variety of activities on medicinal plants, including e.g. ethnobotanical surveys, development of *in situ* conservation strategies (e.g. sacred groves), establishment of herbal folk centres, studies on extraction technologies and medicinal assessments, vegetative propagation for most frequently used species, development of standards for commonly adulterated medications, commodity studies of key species in the market, documentation of indigenous knowledge, education for communities in medicine and conservation, and organization of roundtables and working groups for policy and ethics.

Geographic interest: Principally international, but primarily South and Southeast Asia, with links to Africa and Latin America.

Database: Yes.

Information/resources: The organization publishes the newsletter *IMPNews*.

Funding: The main funding is through IDRC with other contributions from Ford Foundation, IFAD, Philanthropic and Corporate Sponsors. The *International Medicinal Plants Network* is a donor organization which is able to fund the activities of other initiatives.

Contact person: Jason Holley.

Address: International Medicinal Plants Network, International Development Research Centre (IDRC), South Asia Regional Office, 17, Jor Bagh, New Delhi - 110003, India. Tel. (+91) 11 / 4619411 (-12, -13), Fax (+91) 11 / 4622707, e-mail: jason@idrc.ernet.in.

International Council for Medicinal and Aromatic Plants

Global

Status: The International Council for Medicinal and Aromatic Plants (ICMAP) was founded in 1993 as a non-governmental organization with a regular membership.

Objectives:
- to promote a series of World Congresses on Medicinal and Aromatic Plants
- to establish task forces for specific subjects which need attention and improved cooperation
- to publish a newsletter
- to establish an information centre
- to promote knowledge of the use of traditional medicine systems.

Activities: See under objectives.

Geographic interest: World-wide.

Database: None.

Information/resources: *ICMAP Newsletter* is published and international congresses on medicinal and aromatic plants are organized. The first congress was held 1992 in Maastricht and the second will be held in Mendoze, Argentina, in November 1997.

Funding: Funding is exclusively through contributions by members.

Contact person: H. H. van der Borg, Secretary-General.

Address of Secretary-General: H. H. van der Borg, Hijlekamp 11, 6585 XT Mook, The Netherlands, Tel. (+31) 24 / 696-2016, Fax (+31) 24 / 969-2865.

Address: International Council for Medicinal and Aromatic Plants, IUBS, 51 Boulevard de Montmorency, 75016 Paris, France. Telex: ICSU 645554 F, e-mail: iubs@paris7.jussieu.fr.

Global

IUCN / SSC Medicinal Plant Specialist Group

Status: Non-governmental organization belonging to the IUCN Specialist Groups of the Species Survival Commission. At present with 42 members who are appointed by the chair. The group was founded in 1984.

Objective:
- to co-ordinate activities for the sustainable utilization and conservation of medicinal plants throughout the world.

Activities: Activities include assistance in preserving the genetic resources of medicinal plants, the identification of priority taxa and regions for conservation, the promotion of the rational and sustainable utilization of medicinal plants, the assistance of other groups and authorities in the designation and implementation of their own programmes, and the creation of public awareness especially in the resource countries.

Geographic interest: Global.

Database: Database with addresses of personal contacts.

Information/resources: The newsletter *Medicinal Plant Conservation* is published once or twice a year.

Funding: No regular budget. Some activities are supported by the German Federal Agency for Nature Conservation.

Contact persons: Dr. Tony Cunningham and Dr. Uwe Schippmann (chairmen).

Addresses: Dr. Tony Cunningham, P.O. Box 42, Betty's Bay 7141, South Africa (Tel./Fax: 27.2823.29731) and Dr. Uwe Schippmann, Bundesamt für Naturschutz, Konstantinstr. 110, 53179 Bonn. Tel.: (+49) 228 / 9543432, Fax: (+49) 228 / 9543-470.

Global (Tropics)

Rainforest Medical Foundation

Status: Non-governmental organization founded in 1991.

Objective:
- to raise awareness on „Health Consequences of Rainforest Extinction“ with the ultimate goal of helping to save the rainforests and their indigenous peoples.

Activities: A travelling exhibition was assembled that travelled for two years (1992–1994) around the Netherlands and was opened in Paramaribo, Surinam, in 1995. A research project on anti-malarial plants on behalf of the Yanomami Indians of Brazil was supported, and the herbarium collection at Paramaribo is protected with insecticides on a regular basis. A cooperation project is run with two Surinam organizations to increase safety in the use of medicinal plants.

Geographic interest: Tropics.

Database: None.

Information/resources: Bi-annual newsletter, the *Rainforest Medical Bulletin*. Exhibition guide, articles on various journals.

Funding: Mainly private donations. An exhibition was supported by the Dutch Government via IUCN Amsterdam. Requests for the funding of projects by other institutions are brought to the attention of larger funding agencies.

Contact person: Arnould P. van Seters.

Address: Rainforst Medical Foundation (Stichting Rainforst Medical), Einthovenlaan 8, 2105 TJ Heemstede, the Netherlands. Tel.: (+31) 23 / 5280081, Fax: (+31) 23 / 5293483, e-mail: Rainforest@RULFSW.Leidenuniv.NL.

Society for Medicinal Plant Research

Global

Status: Scientific non-governmental organization with a membership of approx. 900. The society was founded as *Deutsche Gesellschaft für Arzneipflanzenforschung und -therapie* in 1953, but subsequently changed its name to *Gesellschaft für Arzneipflanzenforschung (Society for Medicinal Plant Research*.

Objective:

- to advance research and science in the field of medicinal plants.

Activities: Annual congresses are organised in order to improve communication among scientists of various disciplines. Support is given to the journal *Planta Medica: Natural Products and Medicinal Plants Research*. There are cooperative programmes with organizations pursuing similar aims. Grants for research work are provided.

Geographic interest: World-wide.

Database: None.

Information/resources: In addition to the journal *Planta Medica* the *GA Newsletter* is published.

Funding: Membership fees.

Contact person: Prof. Dr. Gerhard Franz.

Address: Society for Medicinal Plant Research, Pharmaceutical Biology, University of Regensburg, 93040 Regensburg, Germany. Tel. (+49) 941 / 94347-61, Fax: (+49) 941 / 94347-62, e-mail: gerhard.franz@chemie.uni-regensburg.de.

Global

TRAFFIC

Status: Joint Programme of World Wide Fund for Nature (WWF) and the World Conservation Union (IUCN).

Objective:

- to monitor the wildlife trade in order to ensure that it is at sustainable levels and in accordance with domestic and international laws and agreements.

Activities: The trade in wild plants (and animals) for medicinal purposes is a priority area of work for TRAFFIC. Current activities of TRAFFIC Europe include an evaluation of the knowledge of the medicinal plants trade and exploitation in Europe through a literature review, and a thorough review of the exploitation of and trade in medicinal plants in a number of European countries that feature as main consumer or producers of medicinal plants. The activities of TRAFFIC East/Southern Africa include a study on the trade of wildlife medicinals in 18 African countries and Madagascar. TRAFFIC Europe (Germany) prepares a study of the international trade of medicinal plants of Indian origin. There are several additional activities on medicinal plants of the other TRAFFIC offices.

Geographic interest: World-wide.

Database: None specifically on medicinal plants.

Information/resources: *Traffic Bulletin*, published three times a year.

Funding: Funds are mainly obtained from WWF and the EU Commission. There is a funding capacity for projects on wildlife trade by other initiatives.

Contact persons: Anne Vanden Bloock, Nina Marshall, Ximena Buitron, Chris Robbins, Chen Hin Keong.

Addresses

Traffic International: 219c Huntingdon Road, Cambridge, CB3 0DL, United Kingdom. Tel. (+44) 1223 / 277427, Fax: (+44) 1223 / 277237. e-mail: traffic@wcmc.org.uk.

Traffic East Asia (regional office): c/o WWF Hong Kong, 1 Tramway Path, GPO Box 12721, Central, Hong Kong. Tel.: (+852) 2526-1001, Ext. 335, Fax: (+852) 2530-0864, e-mail: tea@asiaonline.net.

Traffic East Asia (Japan): 6th Fl. Nihonseimei Akabanebashi Bldg., 3-1-14, Shiba, Minato-ku, 105, Tokyo, Japan. Tel. (+81) 3 / 3769-1716, Fax: (+81) 3 / 3769-1304, e-mail: trafficjapan@twics.com.

Traffic East Asia (Taipei): P.O. Box 7-476, Taipei, Taiwan. Tel.: (+886) 2 / 362-9787, Fax: (+886) 2 / 362-9799, e-mail: treatai@msl.hinet.net.

Traffic Southeast Asia: Locked Bag No. 911, Jln. Sultan PO, 46990 Petaling Jaya, Selangor, Malaysia. Tel./Fax: (+60) 3 / 7947220.

Traffic East/Southern Africa (regional office): c/o Department of National Parks and Wildlife, P.O. Box 30131, Lilongwe 3, Malawi. Tel.: (+265) 743645, Fax: (+265) 743648, e-mail: traffic@unima.wn.apc.org.

Traffic East/Southern Africa (Kenya): c/o IUCN Eastern Africa Regional Office, P.O. Box 68200, Mukoma Road, Langata, Nairobi, Kenya. Tel.: (+254) 2 / 890605, Fax: (+254) 2 / 890471, e-mail: nim@caro.iucn.ch.

Traffic East/Southern Africa (South Africa): c/o Endangered Wildlife Trust, Private Bag xii, Parkview 2122, South Africa. Tel.: (+27) 11 / 486-1102, Fax: (+27) 11 / 486-1506, e-mail: trafficza@global.co.za.

Traffic East/Southern Africa (Tanzania): c/o WWF Country Office, P.O. Box 63117, Dar es Salam, Tanzania. Tel.: (+255) 51 / 22664/28468 Ext. 17, Fax: (+255) 51 / 46232.

Traffic Europe (regional office): Chaussée de Waterloo 608, 1050 Brussels, Belgium. Tel. (+32) 2 / 3438258 or 3438258, Fax (+32) 2 / 3440511 or 3432565.

Traffic Europe (France): 151 Blvd. de la Reine, 78000 Versailles, France. Tel.: (+33) 139242402, Fax: (+33) 139530446.

Traffic Europe (Germany): Hedderichstr. 110, 60591 Frankfurt, Germany. Tel.: (+49) 69 / 60500380, Fax: (+49) 69 / 617221, e-mail: wwfd.melisch@onl.comlink.apc.org.

Traffic Europe (Italy): Via Garigliano 57, 00198 Rome, Italy. Tel. (39) 6 / 844971, Fax: (+39) 6 / 85300612.

Traffic Europe (Netherlands): P.O. Box 7, 3700 AA Zeist, The Netherlands. Tel.: (+31) 30 / 6937307, Fax: (+31) 30 / 6912064, e-mail: jonkman@wwf.nl.

TRAFFIC Europe (Russia): P.O. Box 55, Moscow 125319, Russia. Tel.: (+7) 095 / 2649948, Fax: (+7) 095 / 2649927, e-mail: igor@ch.inv.bio.msu.su.

Traffic India: 172-B Lodi Estate, New Delhi 110003, India. Tel.: (+91) 11 / 4611258, Fax: (+91) 11 / 4626837, e-mail: wwfindel@unv.ernet.in.

Traffic Oceania: GPO Box 528, Sydney NSW 2001, Australia. Tel.: (+61) 2 / 299-6582, Fax: (+61) 2 / 299-6557, e-mail: traffico@peg. pegasus.oz.au.

Traffic USA: 1250 24th Street NW, Washington, D.C. 20037, U.S.A. Tel.: (+1) 202 / 2934800, Fax: (+1) 202 / 7758287, e-mail: Gaski+r%WWFUS@mcimail.com.

Global

UNESCO

See „People and Plants Initiative“ (p. 32).

Global

Wood and Non-Wood Products Utilization Branch of FAO

Status: United Nations Agency. The Wood and Non-Wood Products Utilization Branch belongs to the Forest Division of Food and Agriculture Organization of the United Nations (FAO). FAO was founded in 1945 and has 170 member states.

Objectives:

- to increase the awareness of the importance of Non-Wood Forest products (NWFPs)
- to identify the most relevant issues related to the development of NWFPs sector
- to initiate action to collect relevant information
- to coordinate activities carried out by various public and private organizations in this area.

Activities: The activities are on NWFPs in general, thus including medicinal and aromatic plants, other economically important plants and endangered species.

Geographic interest: World-wide.

Database: None.

Information/resources: The *Non-Wood News* is published on an annual basis.

Funding: The Wood and Non-Wood Products Branch of FAO is funded by member states' contributions. It has the capacity to fund projects of other groups and initiatives.

Contact persons: Dr. A. Gurib-Fakim, Mrs. N. Sufurhally and P. Vantomme.

Addresses: NWFP Officer, Wood and Non-Wood Protucts Utilization Branch, Forest Products Division, FAO, Viale delle Terme di Caracalla, 00100 Rome, Italy. Tel. (+39) 6 / 5225-1, Fax: (+39) 6 / 5225-3152.

WWF Plants Conservation Office

Global

Status: WWF is the largest non-governmental organization (NGO) in the world for the conservation of nature.

Objectives:

- to promote conservation of biodiversity, sustainable use of natural resources and reduction in pollution and waste.

Activities: Activities with medicinal plants include a project on conservation of medicinal plants in Sri Lanka and the general work for the conservation of biodiversity. WWF is, together with UNESCO and the Kew Botanical Garden, a partner in the *People and Plants Initiative* with projects involving medical plants in several countries and working on a number of policy issues.

Geographic interest: World-wide.

Database: A database with contacts in plant conservation was established.

Information/resources: Manuals and discussion papers are issued irregularly.

Funding: Projects are supported by the public, companies and governments.

Contact person: Dr. Alan Hamilton.

Address: World Wide Fund for Nature (U.K.), Plants Conservation Office, Panda House, Weyside Park, Cattleshall Lane, Godalming, Surrey GU7 1XR, United Kingdom. Tel.: (+44) 1483 / 426-444, Fax: (+44) 1483 / 426-409.

Groups with activities on more than one continent

Africa
Latin America

American Botanical Council

Status: The American Botanical Council is a non-governmental organization. It is a non-profit association for herbal education, founded in 1988 by Mark Blumenthal. It is a group with no regular membership.

Objectives:

- to disseminate factual, accurate information on herbs and herbal research
- to increase public awareness and professional knowledge of the historical role and current potential of plants in medicine
- to contribute information to professional and scientific literature that helps establish accurate, credible toxicological and pharmacological data on various types of plants and plant materials
- to promote understanding regarding the importance of preserving native plant populations in temperate and tropical zones
- to provide reprints of plant-related articles, audio/video tapes, and other educational materials
- to assist the Herb Research Foundation in achieving its goals.

Activities: Ethnobotanical surveys have been carried out in Belize, Costa Rica, Peruvian Amazon, and are being prepared for Africa. Mainly pharmacy from the rainforest was studied. Registered pharmacists may receive up to a year's continuing education credits.

Geographic interest: International, with focus on Latin America. Projects are planned for Africa.

Database: None.

Information/resources: The American Botanical Council publishes *Herbalgram*, a quarterly journal. Meetings are held irregularly.

Funding: Funding is by donations. The organization is in a position also to fund projects of other groups.

Contact person: Mark Blumenthal.

Address: American Botanical Council, P.O. Box 201660, Austin, TX 78720, Texas, U.S.A. Tel. (+1) 512 / 331-8868, Fax (+1) 512 / 331-1924.

Africa
Asia
S. America

Chelsea Department of Pharmacy at King's College

Status: Working group at a university. Research on medicinal plants has been carried out since 1990.

Objective:

- to isolate biologically active compounds from plants.

Activities: A wide scope of scientific research include studies on antiviral compounds from plants, plants used in traditional Indian and Chinese medicine (for diabetes, vitiligo and other skin diseases, and for liver diseases), plants used to treat snakebite, alkaloids, biologically-active compounds of the Bignoniaceae (anticancer, antiprotozoal), and analytical methods for phytopharmaceuticals.

Geographic interest: South-east Asia, China, Africa, and South America.

Database: None.

Information/resources: Papers in scientific journals.

Funding: Funds are received from HEFC, various research councils, charities and industry.

Contact person: Dr. P. J. Houghton.

Address: Chelsea Department of Pharmacy, King's College, Manresa Road, London SW3 6LX, United Kingdom. Tel.: (+44) 171 / 3334775, Fax: (+44) 171 / 3515307, e-mail: p.houghton@kcl.ac.uk.

Conservatoire et Jardin Botaniques de la Ville de Genève

Africa
Europe
S. America

Status: University institution, belonging to the Municipality of Geneva (Division of Cultural Affairs).

Objectives:

- to carry out studies on flora, systematics and ethnobotany
- to link floristic studies with sustainable development
- to use the results of these studies in environmental education.

Activities: Ethnobotanical surveys are carried out in several countries of Africa and South America. Enquiries are made among local communities, focussing on traditional uses of plants. This knowledge is systematized taxonomically and inserted in databases for comparative analyses. An important step is the dissemination of this knowledge in terms of education and popularization on a scientific basis. This includes the publication of books, organization of workshops for teachers and others, scientific publications, exhibitions etc. The work covers medicinal plants and also includes other economically important plants such as those used for fiber, woods, dyes, etc.

Geographic interest: Activities on medicinal plants have been carried out in Central Europe (Alps), Africa (Ivory coast, Madagascar), and South America (Paraguay).

Database: Ethnobotanical information received from enquiries is stored in databases.

Information/resources: The scientific journals *Candollea* and *Boissiera* are published and educative materials are produced, including a ducumentary series for the general public.

Funding: Funds are received from the Municipality of Geneva, the Swiss Confederation, the private sector, Swiss development organizations, etc.

Contact person: Didier J. Roguet (Ass. Curator, applied floristics).

Address: Conservatoire et Jardin Botaniques de la Ville de Genève, 1, ch. de Impératrice, Case postale 60, 1292 Chambésy / Genève, Switzerland. Tel.: (+41) 22 / 7326969, Fax: (+41) 22 / 7384597, e-mail: Roguet@CJB.UNIGE.CH.

Samoa
S. Africa

Department of Botany, Brigham Young University

Status: University institute.

Objective:
- to evaluate the medicinal value of plants.

Activities: An ethnobotanical survey is being carried out in Samoa and studies on the pharmaceutical value of lichens are underway in South Africa.

Geographic interest: Samoa and South Africa.

Database: None.

Information/resources: Regular meetings and workshops.

Funding: No information.

Contact person: Dr. Darrell J. Weber.

Address: Brigham Young University, Department of Botany, 285 Widtsoe, Provo, Utah 84602, U.S.A.

Department of Pharmacy of the Swiss Federal Institute of Technology, Zurich

Asia
Europe
S. America

Status: Working group of Prof. Dr. O. Sticher at the Department of Pharmacy of the Eidgenössische Hochschule (ETH) Zurich.

Objectives:

- to screen and isolate natural products and to elucidate their structure
- to develop selective and validated methods for the standardization of medicinal plants and phytomedicines.

Activities: Ethnobotanical fieldwork is being carried out to document the medicinal plants used among the Zapotec Indians in the foothills of the Sierra Juarez de Oaxaca and among Mayan Indians of lowland Yucatan, Mexico. Ethnopharmacological studies of plants used in traditional medicine are made in several countries. Other activities include bioactivity-guided isolation, characterization and structure elucidation of natural products from higher plants and from cyanobacteria, the biological evaluation of natural products, the quality und purity control of phytopharmaceuticals, and the development of selective and validated methods for the standardization of medicinal plants and phytomedicines.

Geographic interest: At present, projects are run in Papua New Guinea, Turkey, Brazil, China and European countries.

Database: None.

Information/resources: Papers in scientific journals.

Funding: Current research projects are carried out in close cooperation with the pharmaceutical industry.

Contact person: Prof. Dr. O. Sticher.

Address: ETH Zurich, Department of Pharmacy, Winterthurer Str. 190, 8057 Zürich, Switzerland. Tel.: (+41) 1 / 2576050, Fax: (+41) 1 / 2625223, e-mail: sticher@phyto.pharma.ethz.ch.

Institut für Botanik und Lebensmittelkunde Wien

Central America
Europe

Status: University institute.

Objectives:

- to educate veterinarians in applied botany, pharmacognosy, plant toxicology and phytotherapy, and agronomists in medicinal and aromatic plant production
- to carry out research in domestication, applied genetics, breeding and quality management of medicinal and aromatic plants
- to study phytotherapy and phytogenic feed activities.

Activities: A current cooperative project with the University of San Carlos de Guatemala, Universidad del Valle de Guatemala and ICTA Guatemala deals with the domestication of several medicinal and aromatic plants indigenous to Guatemala. Applied genetic studies and breeding programmes are carried out for *Achillea millefolium, Amaranthus hybridus, Calendula officinalis, Chamomilla recutita, Gentia lutea, Origanum sp., Papaver somniferum, Petasites hybridus, Salvia officinalis* and others. Special emphasis is put on biodiversity, secondary plant products and agronomic value. Elaboration of guidelines for *Good Agricultural Practice* (GAP) for medicinal and aromatic plants. Use of herbs as diet integrators and feed additives with reference to their antioxidant value.

Geographic interest: Temperate zones of Central Europe (Austria, Germany), Mediterranean countries (Italy, Greece, France, Spain) and tropical regions (Central America).

Database: A database was established on poisonous plants in a veterinary context.

Information/resources: Publications in scientific journals.

Funding: Funds are obtained from research foundations, governmental and non-governmental organizations, and the pharmaceutical and spice industries.

Contact person: Prof. Dr. Chlodwig Franz.

Address: Institut für Botanik und Lebensmittelkunde, Veterinärmedizinische Universität Wien, Josef-Baumann-Gasse 1, 1210 Wien, Austria. Tel.: (+43) 1 / 25077-3101, Fax: (+43) 1 / 25077-3190.

Mexico
Tanzania

Institut für Pharmazeutische Biologie Freiburg

Status: University institute. Research on medicinal plants was initiated in 1985.

Objectives:

- to evaluate indigenous medicinal plants including the ethnobotanical study of such resources, the phytochemical and biological-pharmacological study of selected plants and the study of the sociocultural basis of plant uses
- research on systematics and taxonomy and on phytochemistry of plants.

Activities: Surveys on medicinal plants of indigenous groups are being carried out especially in Tanzania and Mexico. The phytochemistry of selected plant species is being studied as well as the antibacterial, antidiarrhoeal, antiinflammatory and antiparasitic effects of plants used as gastrointestinal or dermatological remedies. Most studies concern the Labiatae and Compositae.

Geographic interest: Mexico and Tanzania.

Database: None.

Information/resources: Student seminars are offered on ethnobotany and related topics.

Funding: Not known.

Contact person: Dr. Michael Heinrich.

Address: Institut für Pharmazeutische Biologie, Albert-Ludwigs-Universität, Schänzlestr. 1, 79104 Freiburg i.Br., Germany. Tel.: (+49) 761 / 203-2806, Fax: (+49) 761 / 203-2803.

Laboratório de Farmacognosia, Lisboa

Portugal
West Africa

Status: University institute within the *Faculdade de Farmácia* of the *Universidade de Lisboa*. A group of approx. 10 persons has been working on medicinal plants since 1984.

Objective:

- to study the chemistry, biological activities and chemotaxonomy of medicinal plants.

Activities: Current activities include an ethnopharmacological survey of medicinal plants used in Guinea Bissau and the study of antimicrobial activities and chemical composition of several African medicinal plant species. Furthermore, the chemical composition of several medicinal plant species endemic to the Azores and Madeira Islands is being compared.

Geographic interest: Portugal, Azores, Madeira Islands, Guinea Bissau, Mozambique.

Database: None.

Information/resources: Scientific publications and regular attendance at congresses.

Funding: University and government funds.

Contact person: Prof. Elsa Teixeira Gomes.

Address: Laboratório de Farmacognosia, Faculdade de Farmácia, Universidade de Lisboa, Av. das Forças Armadas, 1600 Lisboa, Portugal. Tel.: (+351) 1 / 7933064 (ext. 212/213), Fax: (+351) 1 / 7937703.

Africa
S. America

Laboratory of Tropical and Subtropical Agronomy and Ethnobotany, Gent

Status: University institute belonging to the Faculty of Agriculture and Applied Biological Science of the University of Gent.

Objectives:
- to study economically important plants
- to document information on economically important plants
- to educate students in this field.

Activities: Projects include an ethnobotanical survey of the Namib desert with the establishment of a reference herbarium collection and an extensive slide collection. Medicinal plants also played a role in ecological studies in southern Senegal and northern Togo. A project to inventory the ethnobotanical, ethnohistorical, ethnomedical and agroeconomic properties of local and imported food crops and wild species occurring in southern Ecuador is ready for implementation.

Geographic interest: Africa and South America.

Database: Information gained from the ethnobotanic survey of the Namib desert was incorporated into the PHARMEL database.

Information/resources: Research reports and papers in scientific magazines and books.

Funding: Projects are funded by the European Union (EU), the Belgian Government and the private sector.

Contact person: Prof. Dr. Ir. Patrick Van Damme.

Address: Laboratory for Tropical and Subtropical Agronomy and Ethnobotany, Department of Plant Production, Faculty of Agriculture and Applied Biological Sciences, Coupure Links 653, 9000 Ghent, Belgium. Tel.: (+32) 9 / 264-6089, Fax: (+32) 9 / 264-6241, e-mail: Patrick.VanDamme@rug.ac.be

Mediplant: Centre de Recherches sur les Plantes Médicinales et Aromatiques

Burma
Madagascar
Switzerland
Tanzania

Status: MEDIPLANT is a non-governmental organization, founded in 1988 on the initiative of the State of Wallis and the Dalle Molle Foundation. There are four scientific and technical staff.

Objectives:

- to domesticate and breed medicinal and aromatic plants
- to study their chemical compounds.

Activities: Breeding of medicinal plants and research on genetics of secondary metabolites. Research is focussed on the genera *Artemisia, Amica, Echinacea, Hypericum*, and *Rosa*.

Geographic interest: Switzerland, Burma (Myanmar), Tanzania, Madagascar.

Database: None.

Information/resources: Papers in scientific journals and annual activity reports.

Funding: Funds are received from the State of Wallis, the Swiss Federation, industries etc.

Contact person: M. Nicolas Delabays.

Address: MEDIPLANT, Centre des Fougères, 1964 Conthey, Switzerland. Tel. (+41) 27 / 353511, Fax (+41) 27 / 363017, e-mail: joggi_d@gwz.adm.ch.

Africa
Global

People and Plants Initiative

Status: A programme initiated in 1992 by UNESCO (United Nations Educational, Scientific and Cultural Organization), WWF (World Wide Fund for Nature), and the Royal Botanical Garden, Kew (U.K.). The *People and Plants Initiative* is a programme with various projects in the humid tropics.

Objectives:
- to promote conservation and sustainable development through the medium of ethnobotany
- to empower local communities so that they are more fully involved in land planning and land management, related to conservation and development
- to increase the number of ethnobotanists, especially from developing countries, actively working in conservation and sustainable development projects.

Activities: There are currently six projects supported, including: multiple-use management around Rwenzori National Park, Rwanda; sustainable use of wild plants in Bwindi Impenetrable National Park, Uganda; international trade in *Prunus africana* bark; medicinal plants conservation and primary health care in Maputo, Mozambique. A *People and Plants Handbook* is being compiled as a manual on management of biological resources, conservation and community development.

Geographic interest: Although the project has a global approach, all current activities are located in Sub-Saharan Africa.

Database: A database is available with addresses of people to whom references have been sent and who participated in workshops.

Information/resources: Several manuals and working papers have been published, and seminars and workshops are held regularly. *People and Plants Handbook* (see above).

Funding: WWF and UNESCO through national donors (e.g. European Union EU and Overseas Development Agency ODA).

Contact persons: Dr. A. B. Cunningham, Mrs. Alison Hoare and Robert Höft.

Addresses: ● People and Plants Initiative, c/o Dr. A. B. Cunningham, P.O. Box 42, Straight St., Betty's Bay 7141, South Africa. Tel./Fax: (+27) 2823 / 29731. ● UNESCO, Division of Ecological Sciences, 7, place de Fontenoy, 75352 Paris 07 SP / 1, rue Miollis, 75732 Paris Cedex 15, France. Tel.: (+33) 1 / 45684148, Fax (+33) 1 / 40659897, e-mail: r.hoeft@unesco.org. ● People and Plants Initiative, c/o Alison Hoare, Royal Botanic Gardens, Kew, Richmond, Surrey TW9 3AE,

United Kingdom. Tel.: (+44) 181 / 3325771, Fax: (+44) 181 / 3325278, e-mail: A.Hoare@rbgkew.org.uk.

School of Biological Sciences, University of London

S. Africa
SE Asia

Status: University institute. The working group on medicinal plants was established by Dr. D. O. Gray in 1989 and currently includes four people.

Objectives:

- to elucidate and isolate the structure of antifungal and antiviral compounds from medicinal plants.

Activities: Structural elucidations are done with the aid of High Field NMR and mass spectroscopy. For isolation, normal and reverse pulse chromatography (HPLL and T.L.C.), vounter Prolet chromatography and gel permeation chromatography techniques are applied. The efficiency is tested with minimal inhibitory concentrations and cytolovicity.

Geographic interest: South-east Asia and South Africa.

Database: A non-computerized database is available with the chromatographic maps of secondary plant products.

Information/resources: No information.

Funding: Projects are funded by the Royal Geographic Society, National Geographic Society, British Council, and others.

Contact person: Dr. P. W. Grosvenor.

Address: School of Biological Sciences, Queen Mary and Westfield College, University of London, Mile End Road, London E1 4N5, United Kingdom. Tel.: (+44) 181 / 975-5555 (+3018), Fax: (+44) 181 / 983-0973, e-mail: P.W.Grosvenor@QMW.ac.uk.

Africa

Africa:
Kenya
Tanzania
Uganda

East African Herbarium Nairobi

Status: Governmental institution.

Objectives:
- to gather information on indigenous medicinal plants
- to evaluate information on medicinal plants
- to disseminate this information to users.

Activities: The herbarium is mainly involved in the acquisition of ethnobotanical information, especially through the reference material submitted. This information is disseminated to users who need it for conservation, technical processing of compounds, pharmaceutical research, and cultivation.

Geographic interest: Mainly East Africa (Kenya, Uganda and Tanzania).

Database: A non-computerized database (card index) on uses of medicinal plants is held in the herbarium.

Information/resources: Seminars and workshops are held.

Funding: Government funding.

Contact person: Geoffrey M. Mungai (collection manager).

Address: East African Herbarium, P.O. Box 45166, Nairobi, Kenya. Tel. (+254) 2 / 742161 or 742131-4, Fax: (+254) 2 / 741424, e-mail: Biodive@tt.gn.apc.org.

Africa:
E. Africa
W. Africa

International Development Research Centre, Nairobi

Status: IDRC is a Canadian organization with its headquarters in Ottawa. In Nairobi, there is a regional office for eastern and southern Africa.

Objective:
- to fund research activities in developing countries.

Activities: Current projects supported include an inventory and study of medicinal plants of Malawi, propagation and sustainable utilization of medicinal plants in Uganda, conservation of endemic medicinal plants in Madagascar, and the study of *Ocimum* as an anti-malarial plant in Kenya. A project on the use of medicinal plants by local communities of Kenya is ready for implementation and a transnational project (Burkina Faso and Guinea) on biopesticides is being developed.

Geographic interest: Eastern, Western and Southern Africa.

Database: None.

Information/resources: Many publications and meetings on project level.

Funding: Government of Canada.

Contact person: Dr. Serge Dubé (senior programme specialist).

Address: International Development Research Centre, Regional Office for eastern and southern Africa, Liaison House State House Avenue, P.O. Box 62084, Nairobi, Kenya. Tel.: (+254) 2 / 713160-1 and 713355-6, Fax: (+254) 2 / 711063.

Natural Products Research Network for Eastern and Central Africa (NAPRECA)

Africa:
E. Africa
Cent. Africa

Status: Non-governmental network of African natural products researchers of Eastern and Central Africa. Founded in 1984, it now has over 200 members.

Objectives:
- to develop and promote teaching and research in the area of natural products, including chemistry, biology and pharmacology
- to disseminate information to African researchers engaged in natural products research.

Activities: NAPRECA members are national teaching and research institutions and individuals in 8 network member countries. NAPRECA itself does not undertake research, but serves to promote and develop teaching and research. This is done by dissemination of information (newsletter, literature database) and an exchange of researchers scheme, which provides opportunities for scientists, particularly young researchers, to work in selected laboratories in the subregion. The activities cover medicinal plants, plants used in cosmetics, other economically important species (e.g. *Aloe* and essential oil bearing plants), and endangered species.

Geographic interest: Eastern and Central Africa (Ethiopia, Kenya, Madagascar, Sudan, Tanzania, Rwanda, Uganda, and Zimbabwe).

Database: A database of African plants in the current phytochemical literature has been created.

Information/resources: A *NAPRECA Newsletter* (ISSN 1022-3177) is published twice a year and in 1996 is in its 13th year. A monograph series on natural products is published. Symposia on natural products are held once every two years, and summer schools and training workshops on a regular basis.

Funding: Support has been received by UNESCO, Deutscher Akademischer Austauschdienst (DAAD, Germany), International Program in the Chemical Sciences (IPICS, Sweden), and SAREC (Sweden).

Newsletter editor: Dr. Ermias Dagne, Chemistry Department, Addis Ababa University, P.O. Box 1176, Addis Ababa, Ethiopia. Fax (+251) 1 / 552112.

Contact person: Dr. M. H. H. Nkunya (executive secretary).

Address: NAPRECA, Chemistry Department, University of Dar es Salaam, P.O. Box 35061, Dar es Salaam, Tanzania. Fax: (+255) 51 / 43038.

Burkino Faso

Regeneration Sahel

Status: Non-governmental association of approximately 1000 village women. The group was initiated by Joan Zahler in 1995.

Objectives:
- to reverse the general trend of the disappearance of medicinal trees in the Sahelian zone of Burkina Faso
- to further the traditional knowledge in medicinal trees.

Activities: Womens' groups in the region around Barsalogho, Burkina Faso, are organized to plant community plantations of medicinal trees. The women share knowledge of how different tree parts can be used to treat illnesses.

Geographic interest: Central and northern parts of Burkina Faso in the Department of Barsalogho.

Database: None.

Information/resources: None.

Funding: Funds are received from charities and NGOs.

Contact person: Joan Zahler.

Address: Regeneration Zahel, Joan Zahler, 01 B.P. 1265, Ouagadougon 01, Burkina Faso. Tel.: (+226) 367561, Fax: (+226) 360057.

Levla-Levla Group for Agriculture and Environment Acts

Cameroun

Status: Non-governmental company. Founded in 1990 as a sub-group of Dzekwa Farmers Tree Planting Coop. Society, whose objective is agroforestry and afforestation.

Objectives:

- to ensure the availability of medicinal plants for general health care by traditional treatment methods
- to encourage other groups and individuals to run conservation programmes, especially for endangered species of medicinal plants
- to make a link between traditional healers and researchers on medicinal plants
- to purchase medicinal plants.

Activities: Workshops on ethnobotany are held with traditional healers in the Bui area in order to gain a better understanding of the use and distribution of medicinal plants. An education programme is run for the rural population to promote the need for conservation of medicinal plants. Medicinal plants are also grown in a nursery.

Geographic interest: Cameroun (Northwest Province, Bui Division, Jativi Subdivision).

Database: No computerized database.

Information/resources: No information.

Funding: Funded by members. The group has some capacity to fund other initiatives, especially basic medicinal plants conservation groups and projects.

Contact person: Mainimo Christopher Levla.

Address: Levla-Levla Group for Agriculture and Environment Acts, P.O. Box 10, Jahiri-Bui, N.W. Province, Cameroun.

Limbe Botanical Garden & Herbarium, Cameroun

Cameroun

Status: Governmental Botanical Garden established by the German colonial government in 1892.

Objective:

- to promote sustainable utilization of the plants through applied research.

Activities: Ethnobotanical surveys are conducted among local people. The Botanical Garden has a medicinal plants collection, and conservation efforts are made for over-exploited, endangered species through cultivation (ex situ conservation). In addition to medicinal plants, special emphasis is given to food plants, spices, stimulants, and endangered species.

Geographic interest: Cameroun, mainly the Sur Province.

Database: Databases are used for the analyses of field data and the maintenance of living collections.

Information/resources: Brochures and leaflets are produced for dissemination, and workshops and seminars are held regularly.

Funding: The garden management is supported by the Overseas Development Administration (ODA, U.K.)

Contact person: Terry C. H. Sunderland (advisor).

Address: Limbe Botanical Garden, c/o FCO (Douala), King Charles Street, London SW1A 2AH, United Kingdom. Fax: (+44) 1 / 237 / 428896.

Ethiopia

Meftihie Pharmaceutical Enterprise, Addis Ababa

Status: Private, non-governmental company, affiliated to Addis Ababa University. The enterprise was founded 1988 by Dr. Belachew Desta and currently has a staff of seven.

Objectives:
- to collect traditional knowledge on the identity, therapeutic and economic application of medicinal plants
- to determine the toxicity and pharmacological activities of extracts of medicinal plants for the subsequent validation of practical therapeutic effect
- to develop pharmaceutical products for application in health care
- to sell ownership rights of novel and effective pharmaceutical products to international companies
- to cultivate useful medicinal plants, establish herbal gardens and foster the conservation of medicinal plants in their natural habitats.

Activities: The activities encompass ethnobotanical surveys, ethnopharmacology, research on pharmaceutical efficiency and application, technical processing of compounds, cultivation, conservation advocacy, patient consultation, and medication service using novel formulations. Current activities focus on medicines against cold and flu, burns (skin replenishers), heart diseases, hypertension (calcium blockers) etc.

Geographic interest: Ethiopia.

Database: Information on medicinal plants and patient medication profiles is stored in a retrieval system to support medication consultation work and the preparation of publications.

Information/resources: Articles in scientific journals. Seminars and workshops are organized about four times a year.

Funding: The enterprise has received support from the World Health Organization (WHO) from 1978 to 1982 and from the United Nations Development Programme (UNDP) from 1988 to 1996.

Contact person: Dr. Belachew Desta.

Address: Meftihie Pharmaceutical Enterprise, P.O. Box 33121, Addis Ababa, Ethiopia. Tel.: (+251) 1 / 110016, Fax (+251) 1 / 514800.

Department of Botany, University of Ghana

Ghana

Status: Governmental institute, which was founded in 1948 by the former „Government of the Gold Coast" (now: Ghana).

Objective:

- to carry out botanical studies of Ghanaian plants.

Activities: Data are collected on plant uses in Ghana including medicinal plants and other economically important plants (food sources, agro-forestry purposes). Research is carried out into aspects of conservation relevant to the sustainable use of resources.

Geographic interest: Ghana and adjacent areas in West Africa.

Database: No computerized database.

Information/resources: Seminars and workshops are held irregularly and printed materials are issued occasionally.

Funding: Government funds.

Contact person: Prof. A. A. Oteng-Yeboah.

Address: Department of Botany, University of Ghana, P.O. Box 55, Legon (Accra), Ghana. Tel.: (+233) 21 / 75381-357, Fax: (+233) 21 / 500306, e-mail: Balme@ug.gn.apc.org.

Ghana

Faculty of Pharmacy, Kumasi

Status: University institute. The „Dr. Noamesi Laboratory Ltd." at Hohoe is an affiliated enterprise founded in 1977 by Dr. Noamesi, and is supported by the Organization of African Unity Strc.

Objectives:
- to develop scientifically tested herbal drugs based on traditional knowledge
- to preserve, cultivate and document endangered plant species of ethnobotanical importance and to develop a seed bank.

Activities: Surveys in the field of ethnobotany and ethnopharmacology are carried out in order to reveal drugs used by local communities and to make them available to a wider public. The Dr. Noamesi Laboratory has developed commercially available plant-based drugs for the treatment of common tropical diseases such as malaria, microfilaricides and hypertension, infective hepatitis, diabetes etc.

Geographic interest: Ghana.

Database: None.

Information/resources: No information available.

Funding: Government funds for the university institute. The Dr. Noamesi Laboratory is self-financing through private funding.

Contact person: Dr. B. K. Noamesi.

Address: Faculty of Pharmacy, University of Science and Technology, Kumasi, Ghana. Tel.: (+233) 51 / 60071, Fax: (+233) 51 / 60137.

Ghana

Noguchi Memorial Institute, University of Ghana

Status: The *Noguchi Memorial Institute for Medical Research* is part of the University of Ghana. The working group of Dr. Alexander K. Nyarko, founded in 1984, deals with medicinal plants.

Objective:
- to evaluate the pharmacological value of medicinal plants, in particular their efficacy, mechanisms of action and safety to humans.

Activities: The primary activities are pharmacological and toxicological studies of plants that are used by Ghanaians to manage diabetes mellitus, inflammation, hypertension, malaria and HIV chemotherapy.

These studies also aim to understand the mechanisms of actions of the plants. The toxicological aspects of the studies include acute and subchronic toxicity studies of the plants that demonstrate pharmacological activity. Most of the medicinal plants dealt with belong to the families Loganiaceae, Papilionaceae, Balanophoraceae, and Passifloraceae.

Geographic interest: Ghana.

Database: None.

Information/resources: Research results are regularly published in scientific journals. Seminars are held irregularly.

Funding: The institute and its work is supported by local government sources.

Contact person: Dr. Alexander K. Nyarko.

Address: Noguchi Memorial Institute for Medical Research, University of Ghana, P.O. Box 25, Legon, Ghana, Tel. (+233) 21 / 500374, Fax (+233) 21 / 502182, e-mail: noguchi@gha.healthnet.org.

IUCN / SSC Indian Ocean Plants Specialist Group

Indian Ocean

Status: Non-governmental working group of the World Conservation Union's Species Survival Commission (IUCN / SSC). Founded in 1994 by Dr. Wendy Strahm, it now has a regular membership with approx. 25 members.

Objectives:
- to determine and review on a continuity basis the status of native plants in the region of southwest Indian Ocean
- to promote research on plant conservation in this region.

Activities: Current activities concentrate on an inventory of the threatened plants in the region of the Southwest Indian Ocean and include the islands of Seychelles, Comores, Mauritius and Rodrigues.

Geographic interest: Southwest Indian Ocean with emphasis on the Comores, Seychelles and Mascarene Islands.

Database: None.

Information: An annual newsletter is published.

Funding: Various.

Contact person: M. E. Dulloo.

Address: IUCN/SSC Indian Ocean Plants Specialist Group, c/o Mauritian Wildlife Appeal Fund, Wing B, 6th Floor, Ken Lee Building, Edith Cavell Street, Port-Louis, Mauritius. Tel. (+230) 211-1749, Fax (+230) 211-1789.

Kenya

Kenya Forestry Research Institute

Status: Government institute under the Ministry of Research, Science and Technology in 1990. The institute has a present staff of five.

Objectives:
- to collect, evaluate and document local traditional knowledge on medicinal and nutritional indigenous wild plants
- to generate a multi-disciplinary information base on Kenyan medicinal and nutritional wild plants
- to develop a national information resource centre in the area of non-wood forest products.

Activities: The activities include surveys and field identification of medicinal and nutritional plants, the documentation of traditional knowledge on harvesting of plants and preparation of medicines, the propagation of medicinal plants, the dissemination of these plants to selected Traditional Medical Practitioners (TMP), and the establishment of model botanic gardens particularly for the cultivation of over-exploited species.

Geographic interest: Kenya.

Database: Information on Kenyan medicinal and nutritional plants is stored in a computerized database in order to provide baseline information for researchers, foresters, policy makers etc.

Information/resources: No information available.

Funding: Funds are received from the Government of Kenya and the African Academy of Sciences, although funds are inadequate for achieving the objectives.

Contact person: Francis N. Gachathi (plant taxonomist).

Address: Kenya Forestry Research Institute, P.O. Box 20412, Nairobi, Kenya. Tel.: (+254) 154 / 32891/2, 32541, e-mail: Kefri@arcc.permanet.org.

Kenya Woodfuel and Agroforestry Programme (KWAP)

Status: Governmental programme of the Ministry of Energy executed by ETC-Kenya Consultants and funded by the Netherlands International Development Cooperation (DGIS). Implementation started in 1984 as the Kenya Woodfuel Development Programme, and was initiated by the Ministry of Energy and the Netherlands International Development Cooperation (DGIS). KWAP is expected to be terminated in 1998.

Objective:

- to contribute to a sustainable rural production development that responds to the woody biomass needs of the rural household.

Activities: The project has a special interest in medicinal plants. It collects and documents indigenous knowledge, including information on medicinal uses of plants. KWAP creates awareness of the important uses of, mostly, trees and shrub and motivates rural communities to conserve the existing fauna and flora and to increase the tree population on farms. Medicinal plants worked with include *Azadirachta indica, Warburgia ugandensis, Croton megalocarpus, Morus alba*, and *Prunus africana*.

Geographic interest: Western Kenya (Kakamega, Vihiga, Kisii, Nyamira, Busia, Kericho, Migori, and Uasin Gishu Districts).

Database: None specifically on medicinal plants.

Information/resources: Many printed materials on agroforestry and related topics for Extension People and Farmers; survey reports including ethnobotanical reports.

Funding: Funded by the Netherlands International Development Cooperation (DGIS). KWAP has (restricted) capacity to assist in the funding and carrying out of other initiatives.

Contact person: Rik Thijssen (Agroforestry and Farming Systems Expert).

Postal address: Kenya Woodfuel and Agroforestry Programme, c/o ETC-Kenya Consultants, P.O. Box 76378, Nairobi, Kenya. Tel.: (+254) 321 / 63671, Fax: (+254) 321 / 63695.

Physical address: Kenya Woodfuel and Agroforestry Programme, Nandi Road, P.O. Box 9050, Eldoret, Kenya.

Kenya

Nu-Tech Laboratories (NTL), Nairobi

Status: NTL is a non-governmental company run by three directors who work in different institutions with different background. The company was founded in 1994.

Objectives:
- to offer training courses on African complementary medicine, medicine, information on medicinal plants, analytical and medical diagnosis, and study tours
- to offer consultancy services on the evaluation of plant-derived herbal medicines, development of medicinal plant cultivation, identification of medicinal plants, advice on laboratory equipment, and medical diagnosis
- to increase awareness of threats to, and the need for conservation of, medicinal plants worldwide.

Activities: The Nu-Tech Courses in African Indigenous Medicine and Medicinal Plants have the following contents: ethnobotany and plant conservation, identification of medicinal plants, African traditional medicine and its practice, evaluation of traditional medicines, ethnomedical, clinical, pharmacological, toxicological and phytochemical correlations, preparation of herbal medicines, and visits to traditional practitioners and to relevant places of interest. The courses last 3–7 days.

Geographic interest: Kenya.

Database: No computerized database.

Information/resources: Information brochures on activities, seminars and workshops etc.

Funding: Fees for training courses, cooperative projects etc.

Address: Nu-Tech Laboratories, P.O. Box 8014, Nairobi, Kenya. Tel.: (+254) 2 / 214912.

Malawi

Forestry Research Institute of Malawi (FRIM)

Status: The Forestry Research Institute of Malawi is a governmental institute founded in 1957 and belonging to the Forestry Department of the Ministry of Natural Resources.

Objectives:
- to conduct research on forestry and forest products in areas of

silviculture, genetics, seed technology, soils, pathology, entomology, agroforestry, wood and non-wood products including medicinal plants.

Activities: Medicinal plants play an important role in the „Miombo Woodland Management Project". Local communities use medicinal plants for silvicultural systems.

Geographic interest: Malawi.

Database: None specifically on medicinal plants. Information on research trials and seeds is processed with a database.

Information/resources: The FRIM Newsletter is published quarterly. Irregular FRIM reports.

Funding: Government funds. FRIM can support local initiatives and projects on sustainable development.

Contact person: L. A. Sitaubi (Chief Forestry Research Officer).

Address: Forestry Research Institute of Malawi, P.O. Box 270, Zomba, Malawi. Tel.: (+265) 522-866, Fax (+265) 522-782.

Faculty of Science, Mauritius, and Mauritius Research Council

Mauritius

Status: The working group of Dr. A. Gurib-Fakim at the Faculty of Science of the University of Mauritius, in cooperation with the Mauritius Research Council, is dealing with medicinal plants.

Objectives:
- to carry out an inventory of and study on medicinal and aromatic plants of the Islands of Mauritius and Rodrigues
- to study the pharmacological properties of extracts of endemic plants
- to create a database of botanical, phytochemical, physiochemical and ethnobotanical information on the medicinal plants of Mauritius and Rodrigues.

Activities: Activities cover medicinal, aromatic and endangered plants with emphasis on endemic species. Ethnobotanical surveys are being carried out and laboratory research on pharmacological properities is being done.

Geographic interest: Mascarene region of the Indian Ocean with emphasis on the islands of Mauritius and Rogridues.

Database: A computerized database is being developed with the objective of providing an inventory of all medicinal and aromatic plants of Mauritius and Rodrigues along with their distribution, ethnobotany, phytochemistry, physiochemistry etc.

Information/resources: Handbooks on the Medicinal Plants of Mauritius (one volume with 580 pp. published in 1994, two volumes in preparation) and Rodrigues have been published. A large number of articles in scientific journals give information on particular aspects.

Funding: Funds have been granted by the European Union.

Contact persons: Dr. A. Gurib-Fakim and Mrs. N. Sufurhally.

Addresses: Faculty of Science, University of Mauritius, Reduit, Mauritius. Tel. (+230) 4651235 - 38, Fax (+230) 4651239. ● The Mauritius Research Council, Best House, St. Jean Road, Quatre Bornes, Mauritius.

Mauritius

National Parks and Conservation Service Mauritius

Status: The *National Parks and Conservation Service* is a government agency established in 1994.

Objective:
- to manage the Black River Gorges National Parks.

Activities: The organization is involved in the conservation of endemic plants, many of which have medicinal properties. *In situ* conservation is done by creating conservation management areas, *ex situ* conservation through propagation of plants from seeds and vegetation material. Plants are translocated to their original sites. Ecologically damaged offshore islands are being restored.

Geographic interest: Black River Gorges National Park (6,574 ha) and other nature reserves on Mauritius.

Database: Relevant data on all endemic plants is being compiled.

Information/resources: Annual activity reports are produced.

Funding: Funding is through the World Bank and local sources.

Contact persons: Y. Mungroo (director) and Mr. Vishnuduth Bachraz (scientific officer).

Address: National Parks and Conservation Service, Reduit, Mauritius. Tel. (+230) 464-4016, Fax: (+230) 465-1184.

National Institute for Pharmaceutical Research and Development, Abuja

Nigeria

Status: Governmental institute belonging to the *Federal Ministry of Science and Technology* with a staff of approximately 200.

Objectives:
- to carry out research and development work on drugs and pharmaceutical raw materials as well as cosmetics and food supplements from indigenous natural resources
- to evaluate, standardize, purify and preserve medicinal substances so as to establish safety standards and rational utilization of traditional medicines
- to promote environmental science for the improvement of the quality of life and preservation of the ecosystem.

Activities: See under objectives.

Geographic interest: Nigeria.

Database: No information.

Information/resources: No information.

Funding: Government funds.

Contact person: Prof. C. O. N. Wambebe (director).

Address: National Institute for Pharmaceutical Research and Development, Idu Industrial Area, P.M.B. 21, Garki, Abuja, FCT, Nigeria. Tel. (+234) 9 / 5231-602, Fax: (+234) 9 / 5231-043.

Department of Botany, University of Natal

South Africa

Status: University institute founded in 1985 and headed by Prof. J. van Staden.

Objectives:
- to conserve indigenous plants
- to train students in botany
- to carry out ethnobotanical studies
- to develop new drugs.

Activities: An *ex situ* conservation programme with seed and tissue cultures of *Eulophia* sp., *Veltheimia* sp., and *Kniphofia pauciflora* is carried out. *In vitro* investigations for seed propagations have also been made of *Hypoxis* spp., with particular emphasis on *H. colchicifolia*, with a view to provide the pharmaceutical and horticultural industries with an alternate source of supply and to conserve natural populations which are currently harvested. Ethnobotanical studies are performed and tissue cultures (e.g. for the extraction of anti-inflammatory compounds) have been prepared from *Warburgia salutaris* and *Eucomis* sp. A screening programme is being made on Zulu medicinal plants used for headache or against inflammatory diseases for prostaglandin-synthesis inhibitors. Isolation of active compounds from plants with high activity. Similar screening projects are underway with South African algae for the detection and isolation of prostaglandin-synthesis inhibitors.

Geographic interest: South Africa.

Database: None.

Information/resources: Publications in scientific journals.

Funding: Government funding.

Contact person: Prof. J. van Staden (head of Department of Botany) and others.

Address: University of Natal, Pietermaritzburg Centre, Faculty of Science, Department of Biology, Private Bag X01, Scottsville 3209, South Africa. Tel.: (+27) 331 / 260-5130, Fax: (+27) 331 / 2605-897, e-mail: Vanstaden@Botany.unp.ac.za.

South Africa

Department of Botany, University of Transkei

Status: University institute with a staff of five. Founded in 1992 by Dr. R. B. Bhat.

Objectives:
- to prepare an inventory of the plants of the Transkei region of South Africa
- to document the usage of plants in this region.

Activities: Field surveys are carried out to collect plants and information on their usages by local people.

Geographic interest: Eastern Cape, South Africa.

Database: There is a computerized database with the scientific and vernacular names of the plants of the Transkei region.

Information/resources: Publications in international journals.

Funding: University funds.

Contact person: Dr. R. B. Bhat.

Address: Department of Botany, University of Transkei, Private Bag xi, Umtata-5100, South Africa. Tel.: (+27) 471 / 3022811, Fax (+27) 471 / 311666, e-mail: Bhat@getafix.utrac.za.

Institute of Natural Resources, University of Natal

South Africa

Status: Non-governmental university institute with a staff of approximately 30.

Objectives:

- to serve the needs of the community in three areas – teaching, research and „development“ or outreach
- to further the equitable and sustainable use and management of natural resources
- to develop natural resources management.

Activities: The institute's *Indigenous Plant Use Programme* has several activities directly related to medicinal plant conservation. The „Southern Foundation Ethnobotany Programme“ studies the use, sale and conservation of medicinal plants used by Traditional Medicinal Practitioners (TMPs) and Tastafarians in the western Cape, the ethnopharmacology of the tree *Mitragyna stipulosa*, and indigenous fruit species with potential for commercialisation. Within the *Indigenous Plant Cultivation Programme,* the cultivation of indigenous medicinal plants with small-scale farmers through on-farm research is tested and cultivated.

Geographic interest: South Africa.

Database: No information.

Information/resources: The *Indigenous Plant Use Newsletter* is published 2 to 4 timesd a year.

Funding: Clients and donors including support from the private sector.

Contact person: Jenny Mander.

Address: Institute of Natural Resources, University of Natal, 67 St. Patricks Road, Private Bag X01, Scottsville 3209, South Africa. Tel.: (+27) 331 / 46-0796, Fax: (+27) 331 / 46-0895, e-mail: Breen@INR.UNP.AC.ZA and Mander@INR.UNP.AC.ZA.

Traditional Medicines Programme (TRAMED), University of Cape Town

Status: The Traditional Medicines Programme (TRAMED) was established at the Department of Pharmacology of the University of Cape Town by Dr. Nigel Gericke in 1993/94. The working group consists of about 20 persons. TRAMED is a project which will finish in 1997, but it will be continued if funding is obtained.

Objectives:
- to promote the use of safe, effective, high quality „essential" traditional medicines
- to promote the documentation of folk-use of traditional medicines, the scientific validation of these medicines, and the conservation of this natural resource
- to contribute to primary health care through the provision of appropriate information to traditional healers and health professionals
- to support the industrial development of phytopharmaceuticals, as well as new drug development for important African diseases, including tuberculosis, malaria and AIDS
- to contribute to the training of traditional healers by serving as a reference centre and intellectual resource
- to enable all these activities to be established on a firm academic and scientific footing.

Activities: A *Traditional Healers Handbook* is being prepared and will be published in different vernaculars. A *Traditional Medicines Formulary* is being compiled to be used by traditional healers. A laboratory screening programme of plants for anti-malaria activity is being performed and indigenous medicinal plants knowledge is being systematically documented. A database on medicinal plants of southern Africa is being created.

Geographic interest: Southern Africa.

Database: In addition to NPRALERT and PHARMEL databases widely used by TRAMED (see description in the chapter „databases"), the database NORISTAN is used. It was developed by the Hoechst/Noristan company and represents the most comprehensive collection of folk medicinal plant information in South Africa. Information is available on 46,000 folk-use anecdotes and in-house bioactivity assays on some 350 South African plants.

Information/resources: The work of TRAMED is reflected in a large number of scientific papers and contributions to national and international congresses. There are regular workshops with traditional healers.

Funding: TRAMED was established with a grant from the European Union (EU) via Kagiso Trust. Other funds were made available through industry and government research grants. TRAMED is developing a foundation through which the research requirements of the country in this sector can be addressed.

Contact persons: Dr. P. J. Smith (Laboratory Director) and Dr. Taryl Felhaber (Director of Information).

Address: TRAMED, Department of Pharmacology, Faculty of Medicine, University of Cape Town, Observatory 7925, Cape Town, South Africa. Tel.: (+27) 21 / 406-6355, Fax: (+27) 21 / 448-6181. e-mail: psmith@uctgsht.uct.ac.za.

The Union Trading Sudan

Sudan

Status: Non-governmental company founded in 1962.

Objective:
- to improve the quality and to maintain quality standards of goods to be exported.

Activities: Standard specifications are made for various medicinal plants and are then disseminated among farmers, producers and exporters.

Geographic interest: Sudan.

Database: None.

Information/resources: Brochures and leaflets.

Funding: Support was received from FAO and I.T.C.

Contact person: Robert B. Boulos.

Address: The Union Trading Co. Ltd., P.O. Box 685, Plot No. 7, Block 5HE, Mek Nimr Street, Khartoum 11111, Sudan. Tel.: (+249) 11 / 776891 or 780902, Fax: (+249) 11 / 776328 or 451724.

Bazaatusanga Babiri Amalgamated Traditional Herbalists Research Centre

Uganda

Status: A registered company founded 1981 by Ssekiremye E.B.G.M.K. Salongo.

Objectives:
- to grow and process medicinal plants for conservation and trade
- to create a research centre on medicinal herbs and health care clinic.

Activities: The establishment of the research centre is still in its initial phase. Medicinal germplasm plants which are endangered in their natural habitats will be collected and grown on a 35 acre field (*ex situ* conservation). The harvest will be for local use and export. Herbal extracts will be processed and research will be done to combat diseases such as sickle cell, AIDS, TB, and typhoid.

Geographic interest: Uganda.

Database: No computerized database.

Information/resources: There are annual general meetings. Seminars are held regularly and printed information brochures are published.

Funding: Income from the sale of drugs, herbs and agricultural products and also from donations. Seminars and workshops are sponsored by foreign non-governmental organizations. There is some funding capacity for initiatives and projects of other groups.

Address: Ssekiremye E.B.G.M.K. Salongo Bazaatusanga Babiri Amalgamated Traditional Herbalists Research Centre, P.O. Box 2707, Kampala, Uganda. Tel.: (+256) 41 / 533283, Fax: (+256) 41 / 245597.

Uganda

Jamii Tiba Society of Eastern Africa in Uganda

Status: Non-governmental working group with approximately 130 members. It was founded in 1973 in Kenya.

Objectives:
- to promote knowledge and develop the standard of local medicine.

Activities: Village surveys are carried out, in which local medicines in the form of leaves, roots, etc. are collected. Medicinal plants are grown in a garden and the efficiency of medicinal plants is discussed among traditional healers. Indigenous drugs are exhibited at international fairs in neighbouring countries.

Geographic interest: Uganda. The office is situated in Iganga district in the eastern part of the country.

Database: None.

Information/resources: Workshops on local medicines are organized and successful participants are offered further training in Kenya.

Funding: Through the sale of local medicines.

Addresses: Dr. R. M. Nambaga, Chairperson, Jamii Tiba Society of East Africa in Uganda, P.O. Box 400, Iganga, Uganda. Tel.: (+256) 2152. ● Dr. Rehema Nambaga Maliri, P.O. Box 4113, Kampala, Uganda.

Mirror Traditional Healers Medicine Research and Treatment Centre

Uganda

Status: Non-governmental organization with a membership of 16. Founded in 1987.

Objectives:
- to promote the use of traditional medicines in the treatment of human diseases
- to carry out research on medicine quality based on traditional herbs, and improve preparation and safety standards
- to engage in environmental activities which would enhance the harvest of traditional herbs from nature.

Activities: A research programme on traditional medicines is being carried out. Human diseases are treated through traditional medicines.

Geographic interest: Uganda.

Database: The records of patients treated with traditional methods are stored in a non-computerized information base.

Information/resources: No information.

Funding: Consultation fees.

Contact person: Dr. Charles Ocora.

Address: Mirror Traditional Healers Medicine Research and Treatment Centre, P.O. Box 722, Gulu, Uganda.

National Council of Traditional Healers and Herbalists Associations

Uganda

Status: Non-governmental umbrella organization of 46 associations and companies. Founded in 1989.

Objectives:

- to unite all groups and associations of traditional healers and herbalists in Uganda
- to improve communication and collaboration with medical doctors.

Activities: A collaborative research project is being carried out with different therapies using medicinal plants.

Geographic interest: Uganda.

Database: None.

Information/resources: Brochures are printed and regular meetings are held.

Funding: Membership fees.

Contact person: Dr. J. B. Karim Masasizi (secretary general).

Address: National Council of Traditional Healers and Herbalists Association, P.O. Box 7527, Kampala, Uganda. Tel.: (+256)41 / 533590.

Uganda

Natural Chemotherapeutics Research Laboratory, Uganda

Status: Governmental institute. It was founded in 1965 by the Ministry of Health of the Government of Uganda. At present, management is being transferred to the *Uganda Health Research Organisation*. 6–20 researchers work at the institute.

Objectives:

- to study medicinal plants used in traditional medicine in Uganda
- to test the efficiency of medicinal plants.

Activities: Ethnobotanical surveys are carried out in various districts of Uganda. A project covers aspects of preservation of plants used by traditional healers. An education and awareness campaign is run on the value of medicinal plants, and a collection of plants is held at a herbarium.

Geographic interest: Uganda.

Database: None.

Information/resources: Reports on various field surveys are available. Seminars on the utilization of herbal medicines and medicinal plants are held with traditional healers.

Funding: Funding is through the regular government budget and through international research organizations (e.g. IDRC).

Contact persons: Mr. N. K. Mubiru and Mrs. Sophia Apio K.

Address: Natural Chemotherapeutics Research Laboratory, P.O. Box. 4864, Kampala, Uganda. Tel.: (+256) 41 / 250488, Fax: (+256) 41 / 235932. e-mail: ncrl@mukla.gn.apc.org.

Uganda Association for Traditional Medicine Research and Development

Uganda

Status: Non-governmental organization founded in 1978, with a present membership of approximately 4600.

Objectives:
- to treat patients
- to establish treatment centres and traditional medical hospitals.

Activities: On-going research is carried out on medicinal plants and other plants of economical and social importance for future use. All activities are done hand in hand with the Ministry of Health.

Geographic interest: Uganda.

Database: None.

Information/resources: Regular meetings of members.

Funding: No information.

Contact person: Dr. Stanislaus Olowo-Chandirach.

Address: Uganda Association for Traditional Medicine Research and Development, P.O. Box 729, Tororo District, Uganda.

Blair Research Laboratory

Zimbabwe

Status: Governmental institution founded in 1947.

Objective:
- to carry out applied research aimed at finding methods of treating and controlling tropical infections that include schistosomiasis, malaria, AIDS, and microbiological infections.

Activities: A current research project is being carried out on plant molluscicides and the chemical elucidation of their efficiency. Ethnobotanical studies are being made for the identification of medicinal plants for the treatment of schistosomiasis and malaria.

Geographic interest: Zimbabwe.

Database: Literature database for personal use only.

Information/resources: Brochures, technical reports and articles in scientific journals.

Funding: Donor funds.

Contact person: Dr. Jerikias Ndamba.

Address: Blair Research Laboratory, P.O. Box CY 573, Causeway, Harare, Zimbabwe. Tel.: (+263) 4 / 792747.

Zimbabwe

Harare Herbarium and Botanical Garden

Status: Governmental institution, founded in 1902. Staff number: approximately 15.

Objectives:
- to provide identification service of plants to scientists and the public
- to conduct research on plant taxonomy and ethnobotany
- to compile knowledge on conservation techniques for indigenous plants.

Activities: An inventory of useful indigenous plants is being compiled. A research project identifies both modern and traditional conservation techniques for over-exploited plant species. Chemical analyses of medicinal plants is done in cooperation with the University of Zimbabwe.

Geographic interest: Zimbabwe.

Database: No computerized database is available.

Information/resources: The Herbarium and Botanical Garden publishes the magazine *Kirkia (Journal of Botany of Zimbabwe)* and the *Flora Zambesiaca*. Congresses are organized for the *Association for the Taxonomic Study of the Flora of Tropical Africa*.

Funding: Government Funds.

Address: Herbarium and Botanical Garden, Box CY 550, Causeway, Harare, Zimbabwe. Tel.: (+263) 4 / 744170 or 725313, Fax (+263) 4 / 728317.

America

Argentina

Cátedra de Farmacología, Universidad de Buenos Aires

Status: University institution. A project with four persons led by Dr. C. Pérez is working with medicinal plants. The project is expected to be completed in the year 2000.

Objectives:
- to study Argentine folk medicinal plants with antimicrobial activity
- to characterise the pharmacological features of the plants studied.

Activities: See objectives.

Geographic interest: Argentina.

Database: None.

Information/resources: Papers are regularly published in scientific journals.

Funding: The project is funded by the Third World Academy of Sciences.

Contact person: Dr. Christina Pérez.

Address: Dr. Christina Pérez, Cátedra de Farmacología, Facultad de Odontología, Universidad de Buenos Aires, M.T. de Alvear 2142, 11222 Buenos Aires, Argentina. Tel.: (+54) 1 / 961-9080, Fax (+54) 1 / 962-0176.

Bolivia

Fundación Amigos de la Naturaleza

Status: The Fundación Amigos de la Naturaleza is a non-governmental organization founded in 1989. It is linked by agreement with the *Biodiversity, Crop & Food Research Unit* (Mosgiel, New Zealand).

Objective:
- to conserve the Bolivian fauna and flora.

Activities: Medicinal plants form an important component of conservation activities, as they help to fund and to justify conservation. Ethnobotanical research is carried out in Bolivia, with emphasis on two National Parks and Wildlife Reserves. Sustainable harvesting techniques for medicinal plants are developed and commercial outlets and marketing strategies are studied.

Geographic interest: Bolivia, with emphasis on tropical rainforests and dry river valleys.

Database: A database was established for information on species management, utilization of certain species, and distribution data.

Information/resources: Reports are prepared and articles published in various magazines. An ethnobiology course is planned for 1996.

Funding: The work is financed by donations.

Contact person: Stephan Halloy (head of Science Department)

Address: Fundación Amigos de la Naturaleza, Science Department, Casilla 2241, Santa Cruz, Bolivia. Tel.: (+591) 3 / 524921, Fax (+591) 3 / 533389, e-mail: Fan@fan.rds.org.bo.

Centro des Estudos da Religião

Brazil

Status: The Centre of Religious Studies is part of the Sociology Department of the University of São Paulo. The centre was founded in 1975.

Objective:

- to study medicinal plants in popular medicine and Afro-Brazilian religions.

Activities: Ethnobotanical surveys are carried out and research is done on plants identified as being used in popular medicine, in particular in Afro-Brazilian rituals. The pharmaceutical efficiency of these plants, including their biological activity, is studied.

Geographic interest: Brazil, in particular the São Paulo region.

Database: For internal use only.

Information/resources: Regular meetings, workshops and publications.

Funding: No information.

Contact person: Mrs. Maria Thereza Lemos de Arruda Camargo.

Address: Centro de Estudos de Religião (CER), Dept. de Sociologia, University of São Paulo (USP), CX. Postal 8105, CEP 01065-970, São Paulo, Brazil.

Programme Plantas do Nordeste

Brazil

Status: The programme was initiated by the *Royal Botanic Gardens Kew* together with the *Associaçao Plantas de Nordeste* in October 1992.

Objective:

- to contribute to the identification and sustainable use of plant resources in the north-east region of Brazil.

Activities: Plantas do Nordeste combines conservation and improvement of ecosystems with positive socio-economic benefit to the local community. There are currently three lines of research: forage plants, medicinal plants and biodiversity, and bee plants (apiculture) and wood for energy will be added in 1996. Activities specifically on medicinal plants cover their identification and evaluation, and the dissemination of scientifically tested knowledge on traditional medicinal plants.

Geographic interest: North-eastern region of Brazil.

Database: A database has been established to disseminate effectively the accumulated plant information to scientists, research centres, and local communities.

Information/resources: A triannual newsletter is published.

Funding: Funding for Plantas do Nordeste is raised from international and national sources, including companies, governmental bodies, charitable organizations, and private individuals.

Contact person: Karen Pipe-Wolferstan.

Address: Programme Plantas do Nordeste, att.: K. Pipe-Wolferstan, Centre for Economic Botany, Royal Botanic Gardens, Kew, Richmond Surrey TW9 3AE, United Kingdom. Tel.: (+44) 181 / 332-5710, Fax: (+44) 181 / 332-5740, e-mail: K.pipe-wolferstan@rbgkew.org.uk.

Brazil

Universidade Federal do Rio Grande do Sul

Status: This is a working group of some 20 persons around Elaine Elisabetsky at the Depto. Farmacologia of the *Universidade Federal do Rio Grande do Sul*. The group was founded in 1981.

Objectives:

- to create an ethnopharmacological collection
- to evaluate medicinal plants, particularly the psychopharmacological aspects that affect the central nervous system
- to train traditional communities to collect and organize ethnobotanical data
- to further the sustainable development of local communities.

Activities: See under „objectives". In addition, current activities involve assistance to legislation regarding access to genetic resources in Brazil.

Geographic interest: Amazonia, in particular Brazil.

Database: None.

Information: Regular scientific publications, information brochures.

Funding: Funded by the Brazilian Research Council, ONEBELAC, the Rain Forest Alliance and COE.

Contact person: Elaine Elisabetsky.

Address: Elaine Elisabetsky, C.P. 5072 Porto Alegre, 90041-970 Brazil. Tel. / Fax (+55) 51 / 226-7191. e-mail: elisasky@vortex.ufrgs.br.

Brazil

Vitae Civilis - Institute for Development, Environment and Peace

Status: Vitae Civilis is a non-governmental and non-profit organization of approximately 13 volunteers. The group was founded in 1989 on the initiative of *Gemina C. C. Bom* and *Rubens Harry Bom*. Vitae Civilis is an institution for transferring know-how and other services to grassroot groups, trade unions, social movements, NGOs and other interested people.

Objective:

- to support sustainable development, environmental conservation and the achievement of sustainable societies.

Activities: Action-oriented participatory studies on ethnobotany and ethnopharmacy are carried out with traditional communities and rural people in the Atlantic forest region of São Paulo State, especially in the Valley of the Ribeira River. Support is given to the creation and functioning of the „Association of the Harvesters and Producers of Aromatic and Medicinal Plants of the Vale do Ribeira". There is an exchange of experience on ethnobotanical research with the College of Biology of the University of Hanoi, Vietnam.

Geographic interest: Vale do Ribeira in the south of São Paulo State (Brazil).

Database: The database „Jureia Medicinal Plants" has been established for the processing of legislative information.

Information/resources: Meetings, seminars and workshops are held regularly. A large number of technical reports and magazine articles has been prepared.

Funding: Grants and donations are received from national and foreign institutions. The activities on medicinal plants are financed primarily by the Rainforest Alliance, New York.

Address: Vitae Civilis - Institute for Development, Environment and Peace, Caixa Postal 11260, CEP 05422970, São Paulo, Brazil. Tel.: (+55) 11 / 813-0690, Fax: (+55) 11 / 813-1639.

Canada

Canadian Herb Society

Status: Non-governmental organization founded in early 1996.

Objective:

- to meet the needs of all herbal enthusiasts who want to share their knowledge and promote the use and enjoyment of herbs.

Activities: Among the planned activities are regular meetings with informative guest speakers, publication of a quarterly newsletter, and the sponsorship of special events and workshops.

Geographic interest: Canada.

Database: None.

Information/resources: A newsletter is planned to be published.

Funding: Membership fees.

Contact person: Allison McCutcheon.

Address: The Canadian Herb Society, c/o Barbara Fox, VanDusen Botanical Display Garden, 5251 Oak Street, Vancouver, B.C. V6M 4H1, Canada. Tel.: (+1) 604 / 263-9182, Fax: (+1) 604 / 283-9298.

Canada

Centre for Land and Biological Resources Research, Ottawa

Status: Governmental institute founded in 1876. The institute has a staff of approximately 200 and two of them are specifically working on medicinal plants. The centre will be re-organized into a larger centre, to be known as *Eastern Cereals and Oilseeds Research Centre*, in 1996.

Objective:

- to further Canadian agriculture and natural products harvest.

Activities: Information on medicinal plants in Canada (autochthonous wild species and cultivated species) is compiled to develop a strategy for protection and sustainable use. Current emphasis is on *Cannabis*.

Geographic interest: Canada.

Database: To be established.

Information/resources: A book on the medicinal plants of Canada is in press.

Funding: Government funding.

Contact persons: Dr. E. Small and Dr. P. Catling.

Address: Centre for Land and Biological Resources Research, Agriculture & Agri-Food Canada, William Saunders Building, Central Experimental Farm, Ottawa, Ontario, K1A OC6, Canada. Tel.: (+1) 613 / 759-1370, Fax: (+1) 613 / 759-1599, e-mail: SMALLE@EM.AGR.CA.

Save our Saskatchewan Species (SOSS)

Canada

Status: Non-governmental organization founded by Kahee Keane in 1993. Membership is approximately 25.

Objectives:

- to identify unethical harvesting of economically important wild plants
- to establish and promote native gardens to help preserve species
- to retrieve and replant native plant species from land that is to be developed or cultivated.

Activities: Currently making an inventory of several species in order to monitor the input of commercial harvest.

Geographic interest: Saskatchewan (Canada).

Database: None.

Information/resources: A newsletter is published twice a year and workshops and meetings are held regularly.

Funding: Private funds.

Contact person: Kahee Keane and David Howarth.

Address: SOSS - Save our Saskatchewan Species, Box 86, Alvena, Saskatchewan SOK OEO, Canada.

Cent. America:
Dominica
Guyana
Surinam
Fr. Guiana

Floristics Programme of Smithsonian Institution

Status: Governmental Institution.

Objective:

- to further floristic research.

Activities: Floristic studies are carried out in various countries and special emphasis is put on medicinal plants.

Geographic interest: The interest is currently focussed on Dominica and the Guianas (Guyana, Surinam and French Guiana), but has previously also included India and Brazil.

Database: Databases are used for the processing of floristic records.

Information/resources: The journal *Smithsonian Contributions to Botany* and the *Biological Conservation Newsletter* are published regularly. Main contributions are published as books, e.g. *Medicinal Plants of India, Medicinal Plants of Brazil, Medicinal Plants of the Guianas*, and *Useful Plants of Dominica* (author, co-author or editor).

Funding: Federal government funding.

Contact person: Dr. Robert A. DeFilipps.

Address: Department of Botany, Floristic Program, NHB 166, Smithsonian Institution, Washington, D.C. 20560, U.S.A.

Cent. America

Proyecto Olafa / CATIE

Status: Proyecto Olafa is a non-governmental project initiated by CATIE. It was started in 1989 and is expected to be completed in 1998.

Objectives:

- to manage diversified forests
- to develop rural communities.

Activities: Among many other activities, several ethnobotanical studies have been made among different indigenous and non-indigenous communities in Central America. Sustainable harvesting techniques for medicinal plants are being developed.

Geographic interest: Central America.

Database: None.

Information/resources: Technical reports are published in a series. Proceedings on workshops and seminars are available. Topics of congresses and seminars were e.g. medicinal plants domestication, herbariums in Central America, the medicinal potential of *Smilax* spp. etc.

Funding: Funds are received from the governments of Denmark, Sweden and Norway.

Contact person: Rafael Ocampo.

Address: Proyecto Olafa / CATIE, Apdo. 7170, Turrialba, Costa Rica. Tel. (+506) 556-6882, Fax (+506) 556-1421. e-mail: rocampo@computo.catie.ac.cr.

TRAMIL Centroamericana / Enda Caribe

Cent. America Caribbean

Status: Non-governmental working group with approximately 90 members. TRAMIL is an applied research programme initiated in 1984. TRAMIL Centroamericana became a separate branch in 1993.

Objectives:

- to improve and rationalize the application of traditional health practices based on the use of medicinal plants.

Activities: Ethnobotanical researches have been geared specifically towards the Afro-Caribbean population of Central America. Through ethnobotanical surveys (interviews with families), medicinal plants are categorized into three groups: to be investigated (plants on which there is not sufficient information), recommended (plants of proven effectiveness) and toxic (plants or parts which are known to be toxic).

Geographic interest: Central America and Caribbean.

Database: A database of institutions and persons who work with medicinal plants in the Caribbean Region has been created.

Information/resources: Every two years, TRAMIL organizes scientific workshops for the evaluation of plants that are studied. Electronic conferences among TRAMIL members are held. Results are published in books, of which *Farmacopea Caribena* and *Farmacopea Vegetal Caribena* are particularly noteworthy. They are published in English, French, and Spanish. Dissemination material is produced.

Funding: Support received includes that from IDRC (Canada) and a cooperation project with the French Government.

Contact person: Dr. Sonia Lagos-Witte (regional coordinator for Central America and Panama).

Address: TRAMIL Centroamericana, P.O. Box 64, Managua, Nicaragua. Tel.: (+505) 2 / 658311, Fax (+505) 2 / 657283, e-mail: tramilca@nicarao.apc.org.

Chile
Paraguay

Natural Products Chemistry Laboratory at Talca University

Status: University laboratory belonging to the Department of Biological Sciences.

Objectives:
- to study economically important plants
- to train students.

Activities: A current project studies medicinal and food plants used by South American aborigines, and covers phytochemistry, biological activity, and ethnobotanical issues. This project is run by a multi-disciplinary team.

Geographic interest: Chile and Paraguay.

Database: No information.

Information/resources: Various publications.

Funding: The project on ethnobotany is funded by FONDECYT, the Scientific Research Council of Chile.

Contact person: Dr. Guillermo Schmeda-Hirschmann.

Address: Natural Products Chemistry Laboratory, Departamento de Ciencias Biológicas, Universidad de Talca, Casilla 747, Talca, Chile. Fax: (+56) 71 / 200-276 or 200-279, e-mail: schmeda@utalca.cl.

Colombia

Fundación Herencia Verde

Status: Non-governmental organization with a membership of approx. 60. Founded in 1983, this group consists of Colombian professionals. The group is a member of IUCN.

Objectives:
- to develop biodiversity conservation and sustainable development strategies in various communities in Colombia
- to recover and to promote the use of medicinal plants in health and conservation policies as a part of this effort.

Activities: An applied ethnobotanical programme is carried out in the high-Andean village Cota and its neighbour Paramo. With the participation of local institutions, 100 medicinal back gardens have been established and considerable progress has been made with the incorporation of medicinal plants into the formal health service. A medicinal plants promotion programme is run among the black Afrocolombian communities along the Anchicayá River (Buenaventura region) with the aim of recovering traditional knowledge in health care. A similar recovery programme is run among the Ingano Indians from the Upper Caquetá in the Colombian Amazon. In close cooperation with indigenous doctors, a therapeutic ritual hose was constructed, and ritual and medicinal plants have been sown in a certain area of a natural forest. Further activities include the compilation of a national bibliography on medicinal plants, the formulation of policies and the organization of university courses on medicinal plants.

Geographic interest: Colombia.

Database: The group maintains three databases: a geographic information system (GIS), an inventory of the medicinal plants of Colombia, and an up-to-date bibliography (including comments) on Colombian medicinal plants.

Information/resources: The journal *Huellas* is published monthly and the newsletter *Retoños* trimestral. A workshop on medicinal plants (on three levels, with a total of 48 hours) is held at Universidad Javeriana twice a year. Several books have been published.

Funding: Projects carried out by the group are funded by international donations and institutional agreements.

Contact persons: Juan Carlos Riascos (executive director) and Germán Zuluaga Ramírez (coordinator Etnomedicina).

Address: Fundación Herencia Verde, Ul 4a Veste No. 3A-32, El Peñón, Cali-Valle, Colombia, 5.A (postal address: A.A. 32802 Cali, Colombia). Tel.: (+57) 23 / 8808484, Fax: (+57) 23 / 8813257, e-mail: carolina@openway.com.co and pesegura@mafalda.univalle.edu.co.

Farmaya

Guatemala

Status: Private, non-governmental organization and a sub-institution of CEMAT. It was founded on the initiative of Armando Cáceres, Lidia M. Girón and Alfredo Pérez and has a regular membership. The group belongs to the National Commission of Medicinal Plants (CONAPLAMED) and the Iberoamerican Network on Phytopharmaceuticals.

Objectives:

- to detect plants popularly used for the treatment of diseases
- to collect and cultivate medicinal plants with rural micro-entrepreneurs
- to validate experimentally the popularly attributed properities of medicinal plants
- to standardize the processing, extraction and formulation of phytopharmaceuticals
- to encourage legislation for phytopharmaceuticals and introduce these products into national and international markets
- to train and disseminate information on phytotherapy
- to coordinate national and international initiatives for the development of phytopharmaceuticals.

Activities: Current activities include ethnobotanical surveys in six ethinic groups of Guatemala, *in situ* and *ex situ* propagation of native plants, *in vitro* and *in vivo* validation of the efficiency of traditionally used plants, clinical trials, organization and training of medicinal plants producers, and advice to the Ministry of Health on legal aspects of medicinal plants.

Geographic interest: Iberoamerica with emphasis on Guatemala.

Database: Information on ethnobotany and pharmacology is stored in databases, but without on-line access.

Information/resources: Various articles in journals and the publication „Fichas Populares sobre Plantas Medicinales".

Funding: Approximately 70% of the funds are gained from the commercialization of medicinal plants and phytopharmaceuticals. Otherwise there are grants from companies and institutions.

Contact person: Armando Cáceres.

Address: Farmaya, Av. Centroamérica 18-92 zone 1, P.O. Box 1160, Guatemala. Fax: (+502) 2 / 305006, e-mail: farmaya@uvalle.edu.gt.

Guatemala

Herbario del Instituto de Investigaciones de la Universidad del Valle de Guatemala

Status: University institution founded in 1990. Staff approximately 10.

Objectives:

- to maintain and develop a reference collection of the Guatemalan

flora, including medicinal and other economically important plants
- to carry out ethnobotanical surveys, in particular in areas of high endemism of the country
- to support ecological, botanical and pharmaceutical research in the region.

Activities: Current research is focussed on the tropical region of Petén, making an inventory and collection of useful plants, and includes an ecological study of tropical forests. Other biodiversity inventories are being prepared for areas throughout Guatemala, especially in Petén, Sierra de las Minas and adjacent regions. A domestication programme for some medicinal plants is underway for the search of essential oils.

Geographic interest: Mesoamerica region (Costa Rica, Honduras, El Salvador, Guatemala, and southern Mexico), with emphasis on Guatemala.

Database: No on-line database.

Information/resources: The newsletter (boletin informativo) *Red de Herbarios de Mesoamerica y el Caribe* is published in cooperation with the Smithsonian Tropical Research Institute, Panamá. Seminars and workshops on medicinal and halucinogenic plants are held at university and national levels. Several scientific papers specifically on medicinal plants.

Funding: Main funds come from the university. IUCN and CARE support the activities at Petén, and the domestication of medicinal plants is carried out in cooperation with the Austrian Academy of Sciences.

Contact person: Dr. Elfriede Pöll (tropical botanist).

Address: Herbario, Instituto de Investigaciones, Universitat del Valle de Guatemala, Apartado Postal No. 82, 01901, Guatemala. Tel.: (+502) 2 / 380336 (ext. -325 and -326), Fax: (+502) 2 / 380212, e-mail: amacvean@uvg.edu.gt.

Tropenbos Guyana Programme

Guyana

Status: Within the framework of Tropenbos Guyana, there are currently two interdisciplinary Ph.D. projects expected to be finished by 1999. They are being carried out as a joint project with the University of Utrecht.

Objectives:
- to make a complete inventory of the Non-Timber Forest Products (NTFP) in the North-West and Pomeroon region of Guyana

- to identify their uses and their population densities in different forest types.

Activities: Based on a completed study of the medicinal plants of Guyana, all vegetable Non-Timber Forest Products used by local Indians (Carib, Waroo, Arowali) are being inventoried and a field guide with drawings is being prepared. The value of these products for the local economy, their cultural meaning, and the harvesting and management techniques used in their exploitation are assessed.

Geographic interest: Guyana (North-West District and Pomeroon region).

Database: For personal use only.

Information/resources: Ph.D. theses and articles in scientific journals.

Funding: Funding of the Ph.D. project is by the European Community (E.U.).

Contact persons: Drs. Tinde R. van Andel and Drs. Marileen A. Reinders.

Address: Tropenbos Office, 12E Garnett Street, Campbellville, Georgetown, Guyana. Tel./Fax: (+592) 2 / 62846.

Mexico

Jardín Botánico del Instituto de Biología, University of México

Status: The Botanical Garden belongs to the National Autonomous University of Mexico City (Jardín Botánico del Instituto de Biología de la Universidad Nacional Autónoma México). A group of 10 full time ethnobotanists works on medicinal plants.

Objectives:
- to document the medicinal plants used in Mexico, their cultural importance and their commercial use
- to evaluate their medical potential
- to study their chemical compounds

Activities: Ethnobotanical studies are carried out in markets as well as in urban and rural communities of Mexico and the adjacent USA. The usage and trade of medicinal as well as edible plants is documented. Collected plants are evaluated in collaboration with phytochemists. Species found to have an effect on human health are passed on to pharmacologists for further studies. Collaborating institutions include Faculty of Chemistry, Institute of Chemistry, Faculty of Medicine, Institute of Cellular Physiology, Institute of Biomedical Research of

UNAM, and Mexican Institute of Social Security. Medicinal plants are also cultivated in the Botanic Garden

Geographic interest: Mexico, in particular the centre of the country.

Database: Information on economically important plants including medicinal plants is stored in a database.

Information/resources: A CD ROM and a video on the medicinal plants of Mexico has been produced. Research results are regularly published in scientific journals. Herbarium, reference collection and slide collection of medicinal plants.

Funding: Funds are available from the Autonomous University of Mexico and different foundations.

Contact persons: Dr. Robert Bye (senior researcher, director) and M. en C. Ma. Edelmira Linares Mazari (head, public information and education)

Address: Jardin Botánico de la Universidad Nacional Autónoma México, Ciudad Universitaria, Apdo. Post. 70-614, C.P. 04510. México, D.F., Mexico. Tel. (+52) 5 / 622-9047 and 616-1297, Fax (+52) 5 / 622-9046 and 616-2326.

Silphion Project

N. America

Status: The Silphion Project is a voluntary organization with regular membership. It was founded in 1993 by Paula and Alison Denham and currently has approximately 30 members.

Objectives:
- to encourage the conservation of temperate medicinal plants through cultivation
- to provide a reference collection and source of North American plant material for medicinal purposes from cultivated plants
- to promote the conservation of temperate plants used in medicine in Europe.

Activities: The project's activities focus on medicinal plants and other endangered plant species of the eastern forests of North America. A reference collection of North American plants is held at Brackenhurst College, Southwell (Nottingham, U.K.). Cultivation trials including *Caulophyllum, Chamaelirium, Cimicifuga*, and *Hydrastis* are carried out, applying principles of conservation biology to promote and retain the genetic diversity of stocks. A detailed study was made on international conservation legislation and its effects on international trade in medicinal plants.

Geographic interest: Eastern forests of North America.

Database: A computerized database is being developed on medicinal uses and current pharmaceutical research on medicinal plants. Information collected includes habitat preference, population biology, cultivation, and propagation.

Information/resources: Seminars and workshops are held irregularly and a newsletter for members is produced according to demand.

Funding: The project is self-funding and has no funding capacity for other initiatives and projects.

Contact person: Alison Denham.

Address: 66 Victoria Gardens, Horsforth, Leeds, LS18 4PH, United Kingdom. Tel. (+44) 113 / 2583194.

Panama

Center for Pharmacognostic Research on Panamanian Flora

Status: Government university department. The working group on pharmacognosy was founded by Dr. Mahabir Gupta in 1992 and includes some 10 people.

Objectives:

- to carry out research on the isolation and characterization of bioactive molecules from the Panamanian flora
- to evaluate traditional medicinal plants of Panama
- to carry out a quality control of herbal products
- to carry out bioassays and pharmacological evaluations
- to make chemical assessments of local biodiversity
- to train university students to carry out research on medicinal plants.

Activities: Ethnobotanical inventories were compiled for the Kuna, Guaynin and Teribe Indians of Panama. A plant-screening programme was run for the „search for antimalarial, antiamoebic, antimicrobial, molluscicidal, and antimyotic principles from the Panamanian Flora". Research on the medicinal plants of Panama resulted in the isolation of 97 compounds, 37 of them new. The current work also includes a study on the legal aspects of herbal products registration. Emphasis is generally on Rubiaceae.

Geographic interest: Panama.

Database: The MEDFLOR database has been established with information on the ethnobotanical uses of plants.

Information/resources: Numerous technical reports, articles in scientific journals and popular magazines are available. The institute has hosted many international courses, seminars and congresses.

Funding: Most of the funds are received from international organizations and bilateral research agreements.

Contact person: Dr. Mahabir P. Gupta.

Address: Center for Pharmacognostic Research on Panamanian Flora, College of Pharmacy, University of Panama, Estafeta Universitaria, Panama, Republic of Panama. Tel.: (+507) 269-7654/55, Fax: (+507) 2640789, e-mail: mgupta@ancon.up.ac.pa or gupta@pananet.com.

American Society of Pharmacognosy

U.S.A.

Status: Non-governmental organization founded in 1959. It has currently approx. 1000 members.

Objective:

- to bring together men and women dedicated to the promotion, growth, and development not only of pharmacognosy but all aspects of those sciences related to and dealing in natural products.

Activities: Scientific information on natural products is disseminated and exchanged by publication of a journal and a newsletter and by organizing meetings, workshops and annual congresses. Education and research in pharmacognosy is supported and the discipline of pharmacognosy is promoted within the broader scientific community and the general public.

Geographic interest: World-wide approach with most of the members from the United States.

Database: None.

Information/resources: The *Journal of Natural Products* (in cooperation with the American Chemical Society) and a quarterly newsletter (*ASP Newsletter*) are published by the society. Organization of annual congresses and periodic seminars and workshops.

Funding: Membership fees and journal purchase. Graduate and undergraduate research and education can be funded through the activities of the Awards and Funds Committee and the ASP Foundation.

Contact person: Prof. Dr. William J. Keller (Secretary).

Address: The American Society of Pharmacognosy, Secretary, Prof. Dr. William J. Keller, School of Pharmacy, Samford University, Birmingham, Alabama 35229-7027, U.S.A. Tel.: (+1) 205 / 870-2981, Fax: (+) 205 / 870-2088, e-mail: wjkeller@mailbox.samford.edu.

U.S.A.

Center for New Crops and Plant Products, Purdue University

Status: University institution. The Center is housed in the Department of Horticulture.

Objective:
- to encourage research and development in alternative crops.

Activities: Among many other activities, the center has established a research and educational programme in aromatic, spice, and medicinal plants. There are close relations with the Department of Medicinal Chemistry and Pharmacognosy of the same university which is renowned for its contribution to medicinal plant research. Both departments offer graduate programmes on aromatic and medicinal plants and on secondary product metabolism.

Geographic interest: U.S.A.

Database: No information.

Information/resources: Regular publications in journals.

Funding: No information.

Address: Center for New Crops and Plant Products, Department of Horticulture, Purdue University, 1165 Horticulture Building, West Lafayette, Indiana 47907-1165, U.S.A. Tel.: (+1) 317 / 494-1328, Fax: (+1) 317 / 494-0391, e-mail: jim_simon@mailhost.hort.purdue.edu.

U.S.A.

Herb Research Foundation

Status: Non-governmental, non-profit research and educational organization founded on the initiative of Robert S. McCaleb in 1983, with currently approximately 3000 members.

Objectives:
- to improve world health and welfare through herbs
- to encourage and support research into the benefits of herbs

- to serve as a reliable source of information on medicinal plants and herbal products
- to publish and disseminate accurate research information
- to promote the rational, informed use of herbs in preventive medicine
- to support developing countries in their pursuit of rational, cost-effective health care using natural remedies
- to help save undiscovered medicinal plants from extinction.

Activities: The Herb Research Foundation's *Natural Health Care Hotline* provides reliable information on the benefits and use of herbs and nutrients to the public. A programme to help legitimize the use of herbs in preventive medicine in the U.S.A. was launched, a literature information service is offered, international development projects on herb growing are supported.

Geographic interest: Principally world-wide, but with strong emphasis on the U.S.A.

Database: A database is maintained to provide information about medicinal plants to the consumer via a telephone hotline.

Information/resources: The quarterly journal *HerbalGram* is jointly published with the American Botanical Council and the newsletter *Herb Research News*

Funding: About 50% of the funds are received from membership fees, and 50% by research projects.

Contact person: Margaret Blank (Office Manager).

Address: Herb Research Foundation, 1007 Pearl St. Suite 200, Boulder, CO 80302, U.S.A. Tel.: (+1) 303 / 449-2265, Fax: (+1) 303 / 449-7849, e-mail: rmccaleb@herbs.org.

Laboratories for Natural Products, Medicinal & Aromatic Plants, Massachusetts

U.S.A.

Status: University institute with a staff of approximately 25. The laboratories were initiated by L. Craker in 1995.

Objective:

- to promote study and research, and the application of natural products and medicinal & aromatic plants.

Activities: Research, teaching and outreach is done in relation to culture of plant materials, tests for bioactivity, use as antioxidants in food, and application in medicine. A journal and a newsletter are published.

Geographic interest: U.S.A.

Database: A computerized list of world contacts with people working on herbs, spices and medicinal plants is maintained.

Information/resources: The *Journal of Herbs, Spices, and Medicinal Plants* is published quarterly. The newsletter *The Herb, Spice, and Medicinal Plant Digest* appears also four times a year and *The International Directory of Specialists in Herbs, Spices and Medicinal Plants* is published annually.

Funding: Newsletter sales and grants. There is some limited capacity for funding cooperative projects of other initiatives and groups.

Contact person: Lyle E. Craker.

Address: Laboratories for Natural Products, Medicinal & Aromatic Plants, University of Massachusetts, Amherst MA 01003, U.S.A. Tel.: (+1) 413 / 545-2347, Fax: (+1) 413 / 545-3958, e-mail: craker@pssci.umass.edu.

Venezuela

Centro National de Conservacion de Recursos Fitogeneticos

Status: The *Centro National de Conservacion de Recursos Fitogeneticos* is a project of the *Direccion General Sectorial de Informacion Ambiental* at the *Ministerio del Ambiente y de los Recursos Naturales Renovables* (MARNR). The project, on which four people are working, started in 1992 and will be completed in 1996.

Objectives:

- to prepare a Venezuelan medicinal plants inventory
- to establish a germplasm bank through active and base collections.

Activities: Surveys are carried out on the traditional knowledge of Coyagua's medicine men. As a contribution to the conservation of genetic resources, plants with known medicinal value are comparatively cultivated in cold rooms and under field conditions. Work is concentrated on Bromeliaceae, Passifloraceae and Verbenaceae.

Geographic interest: North Carribean region of Venezuela.

Database: Bibliographic database of publications on medicinal plants of Venezuela.

Information: Brochures.

Funding: The project is funded by the ministry *Ministerio del Ambiente y de los Recursos Naturales Renovables* (MARNR).

Contact person: Angele Serra.

Postal address: Centro National de Conservacion de Recursos Fitogeneticos, Apdo. 4661, Maracay 2101-A, Aragua, Venezuela. Fax: (+58) 43 / 831932.

Physical address: Centro National de Conservacion de Recursos Fitogeneticos, Ministerio del Ambiente, Callegón la Ceiba, Vía Ocumare, El Limón, Maracay, Edo. Aragua, Venezuela. Fax (+58) 43 / 831932.

Herbario 'Ovalles', Caracas

Venezuela

Status: University institution. The herbarium belongs to the *Instituto de Investigaciones Farmaceuticas* at the *Facultad de Farmacia* of the *Universidad Central de Venezuela.* A working group around Dr. S. Tillett has been dealing with ethnobotany since 1974, the year when the herbarium was founded.

Objective:
- to further botanical research in Venezuela.

Activities: The herbarium provides facilities for ethnobotanical surveys including e.g. voucher specimens. Most ethnobotanical projects are carried out together with anthropologists, sociologists, and geographers and the herbarium provides the botanical background for these studies.

Geographic interest: Venezuela.

Database: A database on the specimens deposited in the herbarium has been established and efforts are made to establish databases on medicinal and poisonous plants and on ethnobotany.

Information/resources: Several articles in scientific journals and several unpublished theses.

Funding: Funded by the National University.

Contact person: Dr. Stephen S. Tillett.

Address: Dr. Stephen S. Tillett, Herbario 'Ovalles', Facultad de Farmacia, Universidad Central de Venezuela, Apartado 40.109, Caracas 1040 A, Venezuela. – And: Facultad de Farmacia, Universidad Central de Venezuela, 3rd Floor, Ciudad Universitaria, Caracas 1040 A, Venezuela. Tel.: (+58) 2 / 60527-15, Fax: (+58) 2 / 60527-07.

Asia

Bangladesh

Centre for Environmental Research (CER)

Status: University institute founded in 1990 and forming an umbrella organization with seven local non-governmental organizations and approximately 50 herbal practitioners as members.

Objectives:
- to protect the environment and the natural resources, with special emphasis on plants important for medicine and ethnobotany
- to sustainably manage those resources with participatory methods.

Activities: A conservation programme for threatened medicinal plants is run with a participatory approach in north-west Bangladesh. A network for herbal doctors has been established in the region with local NGOs and botany teachers, and a multipurpose agroforestry project with medicinal and ethnobotanically important plants is carried out.

Geographic interest: Bangladesh, in particular the north-west of the country.

Database: For internal use only.

Information/resources: The *Medicinal Plants Conservation* newsletter is published by the institute. Leaflets and handouts are available for the conservation programme. Seminars are held on an annual, workshops on a monthly, basis.

Funding: Contributions from members, sales of products and local and international research grants (Overseas Development Administration / U.K., British Council, International Development Research Centre (IDRC) / Canada).

Contact person: Prof. M. I. Zuberi.

Address: Centre for Environmental Research (CER), Third Science Building, University of Rajshahi, Rajshahi 6205, Bangladesh. Tel.: (+880) 721-2370, Fax: (+880) 286-3057.

China

Institut für pharmazeutische Biologie

Status: University institute with a staff of 8.

Objectives:
- to search for active principles of medicinal plants
- to identify compounds with anti-inflammatory activity
- to analyse and standardize herbal drugs.

Activities: Chinese drugs with anti-inflammatory activity are evaluated and screening is made for constituents with cyclooxygenase and 5-lipoxygenase inhibitory activity. Efforts are made for the standardization and quality control of Chinese herbal drugs. Studies are made on the immunomodulatory activity of *Echinacea* species and suggestions for the standardization of *Echinacea* preparations are made.

Geographic interest: China and Asia in general.

Database: An internet homepage is available.

Information/resources: Regular seminars, workshops and publications.

Funding: University funds, government grants and funds received by private companies and institutions.

Contact person: Prof. Dr. Rudolf Bauer.

Address: Institut für pharmazeutische Biologie, Heinrich-Heine-Universität, Universitätsstr. 1, 40225 Düsseldorf, Germany. Tel.: (+49) 211 / 81-14180, Fax: (+49) 211 / 81-13085, e-mail: bauerr@uni-duesseldorf.de.

Institute of Botany, Beijing

China

Status: Institute of the Chinese Academy of Science, founded in 1950.

Objective:

- to carry out comprehensive botanical studies on the Chinese flora, with medicinal plants being a key research issue.

Activities: The use of medicinal plants is surveyed in southern China and conservation measures are worked out. The chamical features of medicinal plants are characterised and some important species are cultivated.

Geographic interest: South China.

Database: A database on collection material is available.

Information/resources: Some research results are published in Chinese journals.

Funding: Funds are received from the Science Foundation of China.

Contact person: Wang Xianpu.

Address: Institute of Botany, Chinese Academy of Sciences, 141 Xilhimenwai Avenue, Beijing 100044, People's Republic of China. Tel.: (+86) 10 / 8319534, e-mail: Libx5@bepc2,ihep.ac.cn.

China

Institute of Botany, Nanjing

Status: The institute, founded in 1929, belongs to the Chinese Academy of Sciences and the Jiangso Province. It has a staff of some 300. The *Department of Medicinal Plants* has a staff of 23, with 9 of them professors.

Objectives:

- to identify medicinal plants and to establish their efficiency
- to investigate plant resources, in particular utilization, stock improvement, and conservation
- to introduce and acclimatize new medicinal plants.

Activities: The institute has set up an exchange programme of seeds, plants and specimens with over 600 organizations in more than 60 countries. Strong relationships have been established with Missouri Botanical Garden, U.S.A., the Botanical Garden of UBC in Canada, and with the Botanical Garden of Tokyo University, Japan. A study is made of the conservation and regeneration of rare and endangered medicinal plants, folk medicine, and the exploitation of new drug resources. Experiments on the cultivation of some well-known Chinese drugs are carried out, and a comprehensive literature study on Chinese medicine is made. More than 600 taxa of medicinal plants are cultivated in the Botanical Garden.

Geographic interest: Nanjing, Jiangsu province of PR China.

Database: For internal use only.

Information/resources: The magazine *Plant Resources & Environment* is published quarterly. More than 200 papers and books have been published, among them *Icones of Chinese Medicinal Plants*, a 9-volume handbook.

Funding: Almost exclusively government funds.

Contact persons: Prof. He Shan-an and Prof. Pang Zi-jie.

Address: Institute of Botany, Jiangsu Province and Chinese Academy of Sciences, P.O. Box 1435, Nanjing 210014, Jiangsu Province, People's Republic of China. Tel.: (+86) 25 / 4432-033 or 4432-126, Fax: (+86) 25 / 4432-074.

China

Nature Conservation Research and Monitoring Centre of East Asia

Status: Non-governmental organization founded in 1994 on the initiative of Prof. Wang Xianpu and Prof. Li Bosheng.

Objective:
- to establish and manage protected areas.

Activities: The conservation of areas rich in medicinal plants has a high priority. Conservation, cultivation and exploitation of medicinal plants are carried out on the basis of the results of ethnobotanical surveys.

Geographic interest: Tropics and subtropics of China.

Database: No information available.

Information/resources: Brochures and project reports are available in Chinese. Seminars are held regularly.

Funding: Through various channels.

Contact person: Prof. Li Bosheng.

Address: Nature Conservation Research and Monitoring Centre of East Asia, 20 Xiangshannan Road, Haindian Region, Beijing 100093, People's Republic of China. Tel.: (+86) 10 / 2591431, Fax: (+86) 10 / 8319534, e-mail: Libx5@bepcz.ihep.ac.cn.

Arid Forest Research Institute, Jodhpur

India

Status: Institute under the *Indian Council of Forestry Research and Education*, an autonomous council within the *Ministry of Forests and Environment*. Founded in 1988, the institute currently has a staff of approximately 180.

Objectives:
- to conduct research on the problems of arid forests
- to meet the regional forestry needs
- to coordinate forestry research amongst various institutes, NGOs and forest departments.

Activities: A reference garden with medicinal and commercially important plants from arid and semi-arid areas has been established. Surveys are carried out on the medicinal flora of Rajasthan and traditional utilizations, as drugs are studied on the basis of interviews with villagers from various tribal and ethnic groups. An index of medicinal plants along with their properties has been prepared. Attempts have been made to develop awareness among local people about the various uses of medicinal plants by publishing brochures and popular articles. The institute has been identified as the national node of India to work on Neem by the *International Neem Network*.

Geographic interest: The hot, arid areas of India.

Database: An address base of people engaged in forestry research is maintained.

Information/resources: The quarterly *Arid Forest Research Institute (AFRI) Newsletter* and the quarterly *International Neem Newsletter* are published by the institute. Regional research meetings and seminars are held regularly.

Funding: The institute is funded by the Government of India, and financial assistance for the projects is received from international organizations like the World Bank, FAO, and UNDP.

Contact person: R. N. Mishra (director).

Address: Arid Forest Research Institute, P.O. Krishi Mandi, New Pali Road, Bhagat Ki Kothi, Jodhpur 342005 (Raj), India. Tel.: (+91) 291 / 42549, Fax: (+91) 291 / 42549, e-mail: DIR@x400.NICGW.NIC.IN.

India

Centre for Indian Medical Heritage (CIMH)

Status: Autonomous body under the AVR Educational Foundation of Ayurveda, Coimbatore. CIMH was founded in 1993 and officially registered in 1996.

Objectives:
- to undertake surveys, documentation and evaluation of the state of the art of Indian Medical Heritage
- to prepare education material in suitably communicable forms for village communities, school children, lay public and medical professionals
- to help establish a regional network of regional training centres for traditional medicine and primary health care
- to promote activities related to conservation of the natural resources (plant, animal and mineral) which form the resource base of traditional systems of medicine
- to institute fellowships and travel grants for folk practitioners and for other individuals and groups who can contribute to these objectives.

Activities: An ethnomedical information project is carried out and propagation studies on selected medicinal plants are made.

Geographic interest: Western Ghats (South India).

Database: A computerized database on various aspects and domains of the indigenous medical knowledge systems is being developed.

Information/resources: No information.

Funding: Government of India.

Contact person: Dr. S. N. Venugopal (director).

Address: Centre for Indian Medical Heritage, c/o Lok Swasthya Parampara Samvardhan Samithi, P.B. No. 7102, Ayurvedic Trust Complex, Trichy Road, Ramanathapuram, Coimbatore, 641045 Tamil Nadu, India. Tel.: (+91) 422 / 214132 or 216849.

Regional Research Institute of Unani Medicine, Aligarh

India

Status: This institute belongs to the *Central Council for Research in Unani Medicine*, an autonomous body under the Ministry of Health and Family Welfare, Government of India. The group responsible for medicinal plants is the *Survey of Medicinal Plants Unit.*

Objectives:

- to survey, collect and identify medicinal plants in different forest zones of India
- to study distribution, availability, ethnopharmacological uses and threats of medicinal plants
- to cultivate medicinal plants experimentally and in the field
- to maintain a herbarium and an exhibition of medicinal plants and raw drugs for demonstration purposes
- to maintain a herb garden for cultivation of imported herbs and drug crops.

Activities: Since 1971, a series of ethno-botanical explorations have been undertaken in different forest zones of India, collecting over 23,000 specimens in about 140 taxa of medicinal plants. 1700 folk medicine claims of plants were recorded through interviews with tribal herbal medicine men. Based on the field work, a large number of medicinal taxa facing depletion due to their over-exploitation in the Himalayan region have been highlighted and strategies for their conservation and cultivation recommended. In addition, a herbarium, museum and herbal garden are maintained.

Geographic interest: India, in particular the north including the Western Himalaya.

Database: None.

Information/resources: Over 70 research papers and newsletter articles in various scientific journals in India and abroad, and 6 books dealing with medicinal plants survey and conservation issues of different regions of India.

Funding: Government Funds through the Ministry of Health and Family Welfare.

Contact person: Dr. V. K. Singh (survey officer, survey of medicinal plants unit).

Institution's address: Regional Research Institute of Unani Medicine, Survey of Medicinal Plants Unit, Aligarh, 202001 India.

Postal address: Survey of Medicinal Plants Unit, Central Council for Research in Unani Medicine, Department of Botany, Aligarh Muslim University, Aligarh, 202001 India. Tel. (+91) 571 / 20225.

India

Centre for Environmental Management of degraded Ecosystems

Status: University institute. Founded in 1990, the group has at present a staff of 10.

Objectives:

- to prepare inventories and to monitor biodiversity
- to study the conservation biology of endangered plants, including medicinal plants
- to develop restoration techniquesa for degraded ecosystems
- to further the sustainable use of genetic resources.

Activities: The conservation biology of *Coptis teeta*, an endangered species endemic to Arumachal Pradesh (India), has been investigated. An agronomic package has been developed for its cultivation and exploitation. A study of the conservation biology of another 11 species of *Meconopsis* endemic to Sikkim (Himalaya) included tissue cultures for propagation. An inventory of little-known medicinal plants from north-eastern India and a monitoring programme is carried out.

Geographic interest: Indian subcontinent (India, Bhutan, and Nepal).

Database: None.

Information/resources: No information available.

Funding: Government funding.

Contact person: C. R. Babu (director).

Address: Centre for Environmental Management of Degraded Ecosystems, University of Delhi, South Campus, Benito Juarez Road, New Delhi, 110021 India.

College of Forestry, Bangalore

India

Status: University department, existing since 1976.

Objectives:

- to survey for wild plant genetic resources from tropical forests of South India
- to develop suitable propagation techniques for rare and important medicinal plants
- to develop *ex situ* facilities for conservation of medicinal plants
- to introduce new medicinal plants into cultivation
- to produce technical inputs to governmental and non-governmental bodies dealing with medicinal plants.

Activities: Projects have been carried out on the exploration of plants of horticultural importance from natural forests in Tumkur District (South India), on *in situ* conservation of medicinal plants at B.R. Hills in Mysore District (South India) and on the development of propagation techniques for rare plants from Coorg District (South India).

Geographic interest: Karnataka region, South India.

Database: None.

Information/resources: Pamphlets are issued, and seminars are held when required.

Funding: The College of Forestry is funded by the government; no external sources are available.

Contact person: C. G. Kushalappa.

Address: College of Forestry, University of Agricultural Sciences, Bangalore, 560065 India. Tel. (+91) 80 / 3330153, Fax (+91) 80 / 3330277.

Department of Botany, Tirupati

India

Status: The Department of Botany is a sub-institution of the Arts College of Sri Venkateswara University in Tirupati. A working programme on medicinal plants was established in 1994 by *IDRC Medicinal Plant Network, South Asia Region*, New Delhi.

Objectives:

- to collect information on herbal potential and folk medicine of the villagers and tribes
- to further *ex situ* conservation of threatened medicinal plants
- to collect information on ethnomedicine in order to further the development of new drugs.

Activities: A comprehensive survey of Chittoor District, Andhra Pradesh, was carried out. Ethnobotanical information has been gathered. Medicinal plants identified as rare and endangered are cultivated.

Geographic interest: Andhra Pradesh District in India.

Database: None.

Information/resources: Articles in scientific journals.

Funding: Funds are received from IDRC Medicinal Plant Network, South Asia Region.

Contact person: Dr. S. Vedavathi.

Address: Department of Botany, S.V. Arts College, Sri Venkateswara University, B-23, Vaikuntapuram, M.R. Palli, Tirupati, 517502 India. Tel.: (+91) 8574 / 21605.

India

Non-wood Forest Products Division at Forest Research Institute, Dehra Dun

Status: A division of Forest Research Institute within the Indian Council of Forestry Research and Education, Dehra Dun. The division started in 1906 and the non-wood division has a staff of 10 researchers and assistants.

Objectives:

- to preserve rare and endangered medicinal and aromatic plants
- to develop cultural practices of medicinal and aromatic plants
- to extent cultivation technologies to farmers, hill communities, government agencies and NGO's.

Activities: A herbal garden and nurseries have been established at Dehradun for tropical and subtropical and at Chakrata for temperate and alpine medicinal and aromatic plants. Methods for cultivation and harvesting medicinal and aromatic plants are developed and disseminated. Surveys are conducted to assess the availability and status of medicinal and aromatic plants in the Himalayas.

Geographic interest: India with emphasis on Jammu and Kashmir, Himachal Pradesh, Punjab, Haryana, and Hills of Uttar Pradesh.

Database: Efforts are made to establish a national database on non-wod forest products.

Information/resources: Regular seminars and workshops.

Funding: Mainly funded by internal and external projects.

Contact persons: G. S. Rawat (head) and Dr. A. K. Sharma (scientist).

Address: Forest Research Institute, Non-wood Forest Products Division, P.O. New Forest, Dehra Dun, 248006 India. Tel.: (+91) 135 / 626847, Fax: (+91) 135 / 626865 or 628571.

French Institute, Pondicherry

India

Status: Foreign institution under French Ministry of External Affairs. The institute was founded in 1954 and is working within the framework of the Indo-French treaty of 1954.

Objectives:
- to map the vegetation of the Western Ghats
- to prepare an atlas of arborescent species of the Western Ghats
- to study the biodiversity of the Western Ghats.

Activities: A programme on the conservation of medicinal plants is run. Their distribution is mapped using a geographical information system (GIS). A database on the ecology of selected medicinal plants is maintained. The institute also holds a herbarium with 4000 species and 30,000 specimens.

Geographic interest: Southern India.

Database: On the ecology of selected medicinal plant species.

Information/resources: Articles in magazines.

Funding: French Ministry of Foreign Affairs.

Contact person: Dr. B. R. Ramesh.

Address: French Institute, P.B. 22, St. Louis Street, Pondicherry 605001, India. Tel.: (+91) 413 / 34170 or 34168, Fax: (+91) 413 / 39534.

India (Himalaya)

High Altitude Plant Physiology Research Centre

Status: The Research Centre was founded in 1979 on the initiative of Prof. A. N. Purohit, as an institute within the *H. N. B. Garhwal University*. Approximately 30 people are employed at present.

Objectives:
- to survey the natural and cultivated vegetation and its use and misuse along an altitudinal gradient
- to study the use of mountain plants
- to conserve *in situ* and to propagate *ex situ* endangered plants
- to study agroforestry and energy farming
- to develop linkage programmes with institutions and laboratories in India and abroad working on similar lines.

Activities: Surveys of economically important plants are being carried out. Techniques for domestication and multiplication of some important, highly exploited medicinal herbs and trees are currently developed and germplasm collections of these plants are made.

Geographic interest: Central Himalaya, India.

Database: An inventory of mountain plants is being developed.

Information/resources: Research papers are available in scientific journals, and seminars and workshops are held at the institute.

Funding: Grants are received from the Government of India and other funding bodies. The Research Centre has no funds to provide for other organizations.

Address: High Altitude Plant Physiology Research Centre, H. N. B. Garhwal University, P.O. Box 14, Srinagar Garhwal (U.P.), India. Tel. (+91) 1388 / 2172, Fax (+91) 1388 / 2061 or 2072.

India

Horticultural Experiments and Training Centre, Chaubattia

Status: The centre was founded in 1932 and belongs to the Uttar Pradesh Government. It currently has a staff of approximately 25.

Objectives:
- to survey, collect and identify medicinal plants in the Uttar Pradesh area
- to develop agri-horticultural techniques for medicinal plants

- to provide training for growers and farmers in the cultivation of medicinal plants
- to make chemical analyses of important medicinal plants.

Activities: Ethnobotanical studies are made in the hills of Uttar Pradesh. A conservation project is run for some rare medicinal plants, and some medicinal plants which may have economic potential are cultivated.

Geographic interest: Garhwal and Kumaun region of Uttar Pradesh (India).

Database: None.

Information/resources: Regular publications in scientific journals.

Funding: Uttar Pradesh Government.

Contact person: Dr. Harish Singh Bhujwan.

Address: Horticultural Experiments and Training Centre, Drug Section, Chaubattia (Ranikhet), Almora, Uttar Pradesh, Pin 263651 (U.P.), India. Tel.: (+91) 5966 / 2221 and 2242.

Institute of Rain & Moist Deciduous Forests Research, Jorhat

India

Status: Autonomous Institute under the Indian Council of Forestry Research and Education. It was founded in 1988 under the Ministry of Environment and by the Government of India.

Objective:
- to identify the forest plant species with medicinal value and to isolate the active medicinal compounds.

Activities: Some plants known in local ethnomedicine are screened phytochemically, their biological activity is screened and their active ingredients are isolated and partially characterised. In addition to medicinal plants, oil-bearing plants and food plants are studied:

Geographic interest: North-eastern region of India.

Database: None.

Information/resources: No information available.

Funding: Grants from the Indian Council of Forestry Research and Education (ICFRE), a Government of India body.

Contact persons: S. N. Kalita (director) and Dr. R. Sett (scientist).

Address: Institute of Rain and Moist Deciduous Forest Research, Naali, Bongal Pukhuri, P:O. Jorhat 785001, Assam, India. Tel.: (+912) 376 / 322-052 or 322-054, Fax: (+91) 376 / 323-895.

India

Lok Swasthya Parampara Samvardhan Samithi

Status: A network of various non-governmental organizations, founded in 1985. There is a membership of approximately 1200, with over 200 being active members.

Objectives:
- to revitalize local health traditions
- to protect regional medicinal plant species
- to create medicinal plant packages for primary health care
- to create a database of medicinal plants.

Activities: A nursery for medicinal plants is maintained. Educational materials on medicinal plants are produced and disseminated to voluntary groups. A database with information on medicinal plants is operated.

Geographic interest: India.

Database: A database with information on medicinal plants has been established for students and interested NGOs.

Information/resources: A newsletter is distributed, and seminars and workshops are held.

Funding: Indian Government funds.

Address: Lok Swasthya Parampara Samvardhan Samithi, P.B. 7102, Ayurvedic Trust Complex, Ramanathapuram, Coimbatore, 641045 India. Tel.: (+91) 422 / 213188, Fax (+91) 422 / 214953.

India

Medplan Conservatory Society

Status: Non-governmental organization founded in 1995.

Objective:
- to support the conservation of medicinal plants.

Activities: A medicinal plants conservation magazine is published. Literature on the conservation of medicinal plants is sold to interested people and a translating capacity of resource persons for plant names (English, vernacular names) is being developed.

Geographic interest: India.

Database: A database for information on education and published information on medicinal plants is being developed.

Information/resources: A newsletter, posters, brochures, and educational materials are published.

Contact person: Vinay Tandon.

Address: Medplan Conservatory Society, No. 8, I. Floor, IV Main, II Stage, MSH Colony, Anandnagar, Bangalore 560024, India. Tel.: (+91) 8080 / 3336909-35, Fax: (+91) 80 / 3334167.

National Council of Development and Communication

India

Status: Non-governmental organization with a membership over 200. Founded in 1983.

Objectives:
- to increase rural prosperity by modern techniques and appropriate technologies
- to act as a clearing house for science and information dissemination
- to gather, process, store and disseminate traditional knowledge and technologies, in particular in the areas of agriculture, environment, health
- to plan and execute programmes related to sustainable development of society through people's participation.

Activities: Among various activities to further sustainable development, medicinal plants play a major role. A detailed field survey was undertaken of the Naugarh Forest near Varanasi within the framework of the project „Participatory environment management". 150 herbs were identified which are being used by local inhabitants for human and animal health care. Based on these results, a project has been prepared to provide health care to local inhabitants. Joint activities with *Ayurved Faculty of Banaras Hindu University* within this project include conservation, multiplication and processing of medicinal plants.

Geographic interest: India, in particular the Bindhyan range.

Database: None.

Information/resources: The journal *Interaction* and annual activity reports are published. Seminars are held on a bi-annual basis.

Funding: Through donations, grants and membership fees.

Contact person: Prof. V. K. Dubey (Secretary).

Address: National Council of Development and Communication, H.Q. B 33/14-22, Koshlesh Nagar Colony, Nariya, Varanasi, 221005 India. Tel. (+91) 542 / 313-700 or 311-974, Fax: (+91) 542 / 313-700.

India

Native Medicare Charitable Trust (NMCT)

Status: NMCT is a non-governmental organization with approximately 80 members. It was founded in 1988 by A. S. Sankara Narayanan.

Objectives:

- to propagate traditional systems of medicines through modern thought
- to conserve the genetic resources of medicinal plants and those employed by the aborigines and other rural peoples
- to develop health oriented development programmes and to establish training centres
- to establish educational institutions and research centres in the various disciplines of traditional practices
- to establish cooperation with national and international organizations with common objectives.

Activities: NMCT is assisting villages to become self-supporting in health care by distributing a package of medicinal herbs that can be easily processed. NMCT has a herbal nursery where traditional medicines are prepared and demonstrated. The herbary includes a collection of endangered and rare plants. Various programmes deal with environmental awareness building and conservation of genetic resources. Consultancy services are offered to any organization.

Geographic interest: Southern India, in particular the Attappady Valley of the Western Ghats and rural villages of the Coimbatore District.

Database: No computerized database.

Information/resources: Regular seminars and workshops on different topics are held.

Funding: Donations from farmers, businesses and trusts. Funds are occasionally received from Government Departments and other NGOs for specific activities.

Contact person: A. S. Sankara Narayanan.

Address: Native Medicare Charitable Trust, 2/232 Somayanoor, Thadagam (via), Coimbatore, India 641108. Tel.: (+91) 422 / 858349.

G. B. Pant Institute of Himalayan Environment and Development

India (Himalaya)

Status: This is an autonomous institute of the Ministry of Environment and Forests (Government of India), founded in 1988. About 30 scientists are currently working there.

Objectives:
- to undertake in-depth research and development studies on environmental problems in Himalaya
- to identify and strengthen local perceptions of the environment
- to evolve and demonstrate suitable technology for sustainable development of the region.

Activities: A core group of the institute works on the conservation of biodiversity. Its activities are focussed on threatened medicinal and other economically important plant taxa of the Central Himalaya. An inventory of existing bioresources including medicinal plants and ethnomedicinal knowledge is being prepared, gene banks (herbal gardens) are established and threats to plants are assessed.

Geographic interest: Himalaya (India).

Database: No computerized database.

Information/resources: In addition to various institute publications, the newsletter *Himaparyavaran* (ISSN 0970-8421) is published by the institute. There are frequently seminars and workshops on different topics.

Funding: Indian government funds and international organizations.

Contact person: Dr. Uppeandra Dhar.

Address: G. B. Pant Institute of Himalayan Environment and Development, Kosi, Almora, 263643 India. Tel.: (+91) 5962 / 81111 or 81144, Fax: (+91) 5962) 22100, e-mail: GBPIHED@SHAKTI.ncst.in.

India

Rapinat Herbarium & Anglade Institute Working Group

Status: This is a working group between the Rapinat Herbarium at Tiruchirapalli and the Anglade Institute of Natural History at Kodaikanal. It was initiated in 1970 by K. M. Matthew and has approx. 20 members.

Objectives:
- to carry out taxonomic research on medicinal and endangered plants
- to carry out a public awareness programme for the conservation of local plants
- *in situ* and *ex situ* conservation of endangered plant species.

Activities: The activities on plant preservation are confined to the Kodaikanal region, where a 3-years public awareness programme is being carried out.

Geographic interest: Kodaikanal region of India.

Database: None.

Information: The newsletter *Shola* is produced twice a year and a number of scientific papers and books are available.

Funding: Both institutions are under Jesuit management and projects are funded through their own budget.

Contact person: K. M. Matthew (director).

Address for correspondence: The Rapinat Herbarium, St. Joseph's College, Tiruchirapalli 620002, India. Tel. (+91) 0431 / 29052, Fax (+91) 0431 / 23940.

Address of field station: The Anglade Institute of Natural History, Sacred Heart College, Shembaganur, Kodaikanal 624104, India. Tel. (+91) 4542 / 41101.

India

Regional Research Laboratory, Jammu

Status: Governmental research institute, belonging to the *Council of Scientific and Industrial Research*. The institute has a biodiversity unit headed by Dr. M. K. Kaul.

Objectives:
- to further the sustainable use of medicinal plant resources

- to protect endangered medicinal plants
- to carry out studies on ethnobotany
- to develop new drugs and natural products
- to take care of quality control and standardization of certain drugs
- to make toxicity studies of selected traditional drugs.

Activities: See objectives. Ethnobotanical studies are made in north-west Himalaya and Trans-Himalaya. Studies on the diversity and conservation needs of threatened medicinal plants are made in Western Himalaya and experiments are carried out on the domestication and cultivation of medicinal plants. In addition to medicinal plants, work is also done on plants used in cosmetics, aromatic plants, food plants, and other economically important plants.

Geographic interest: North-west Himalaya (India), i.e. temperate and cold arid regions.

Database: No computerized database.

Information/resources: The *Regional Research Laboratory Newsletter* is published quarterly.

Funding: No information available.

Contact persons: Prof. S. S. Handa (director) and Dr. M. K. Kaul (senior scientist).

Address: Regional Research Laboratory, Jammu 180001, India.

Tropical Botanic Garden and Research Institute, Karimancode

India

Status: Governmental institution with a staff of approximately 250. The institution was founded in 1979 by Prof. Dr. A. Abraham.

Objectives:
- to conserve tropical plant genetic resources and to develop strategies for their sustainable use
- to carry out botanical, chemical and medicinal research for plant improvement and utilization
- to organize germplasm collections of economically important plants, especially medicinal and aromatic plants
- to act as an all-Indian coordination centre for research projects on ethnobiology.

Activities: *Ex situ* conservation of various tropical plants is carried out, for example, with the establishment of a national gene bank of medicinal and aromatic plants, with root cultures, and through micropropagation of rare and endangered medicinal plants. Various research projects on ethnobiology are organized. Medicinal plants are screened for the detection and isolation of active compounds. Ethnopharmacological studies aim in particular at the detection of antibacterial and antifungal activities, and antimicrobial and pesticidal compounds were successfully isolated from wild mushrooms. Biodiversity is evaluated through bioprospecting.

Geographic interest: India: Western Ghats, and warm, humid, tropical India.

Database: National database on ethnobiology and ethnomedicine, for documentation and utilization for scientific, developmental and industrial purposes.

Information/resources: The *Tropical Botanic Garden and Research Institute* (TBGRI) Newsletter is published twice a year. In addition, leaflets, brochures, books and booklets are available for distribution. Three to four seminars and one congress are held per year.

Funding: Funds are received from the Government of Kerala and the Government of India.

Contact persons: Dr. P. Pushpangadan (director) and P. J. Mathew (scientist).

Address: Tropical Botanic Garden and Research Institute, Karimancode, Pacha-Palode, Thiruvananthapuram, 695562 Kerala India. Tel.: (+91) 472 / 84-236 or 84-226, Fax (+91) 471 / 431-178.

India

Yuva

Status: A non-governmental working group of 6 volunteers. It was founded in 1985 by V. J. Raghuvanshi.

Objectives:
- to develop rural communities
- to undertake programmes in particular for the poorest classes.

Activities: The activities include 3-day training courses for youth leaders to identify local herbs and to learn their usages. A similar one-day programme was offered to 17 different High Schools in Dehgam Taluka and an exhibition of medicinal plants was prepared and shown at different High Schools.

Geographic interest: Rural areas of Ahmedabad District in India.

Database: None.

Information: Meetings are held irregularly.

Funding: No information.

Contact person: V. J. Raghuyanshi (trustee).

Address: Yuva, 8 Bhagyalaxmi Society, Nava Vadaj, Ahmedabad 380013, India. Tel. (+91) 79 / 7450615.

Tropical Forest Medicinal Plant Programme in Indonesia

Status: University project, run by the Faculty of Forestry of Bogor Agricultural University in close collaboration with the non-governmental organization LATIN (Lembaga Alam Tropika Indonesia, the Indonesian Tropical Institute). The project started in 1992 on the initiative of Ir Ervizal Zuhud and is expected to be completed in 1998.

Objectives:
- to promote the value of forest products by developing non-wood forest products in the form of medicinal raw materials, through a programme of conservation of medicinal plants from Indonesian tropical forests
- to explore the potential of forest resources which have not yet been utilized as medicinal raw materials for national development in the field of health or for export
- to increase the income/welfare of people living close to forests by promoting traditional medicine utilization
- to conserve the diversity of germ plasm of medicinal plants in forests
- to screen forest products for new medicinal plants to cure recent diseases (cancer, AIDS, etc.).

Activities: See objectives. A technical guide book for the conservation of medicinal plants harvested from tropical forests is prepared. Another book is prepared with technical advice on the cultivation of some medicinal plants which have a high economic value. A database with information on medicinal plants in tropical forests has been established. Efforts are made to develop new and reliable medicinal raw materials and toxins. In addition to medicinal plants, the programme also deals with edible and ornamental plants and other economically important species.

Geographic interest: Tropical rainforests in Indonesia (Java, Sumatra and Kalimantan).

Database: A database on medicinal plants from tropical forests will be established.

Information/resources: The *APINMAP Newsletter* and the journal *Media Konservasi, Indonesian Medicinal Plant* are published. Seminars are held twice a year, and also irregular congresses.

Funding: The project is supported by the MacArthur Foundation, U.S.A.

Contact person: Ir Ervizal A. M. Zuhud (P.O. Box 168, Bogor, Indonesia).

Address: Tropical Forest Medicinal Programme, Laboratory of Plant Conservation, Department of Forest Resource Conservation, Faculty of Forestry, Bogor Agricultural University, Kampus IPB Darmaga, P.O. Box 168, Bogor 16001, Indonesia. Tel.: (+62) 251 / 621-562, Fax: (+62) 251 / 621-562 or 621-256, e-mail: amzu@indo.net.id.

Nepal

Himalayan Ayurveda Research Institute

Status: The research institute is a non-governmental organization with a regular membership of approx. 30. It was founded in 1994 by Prof. L. M. Singh.

Objectives:

- to create awareness about the conservation of medicinal plants and other resource materials of Ayurveda in Nepal
- to create awareness about the economic potential that medicinal plants represent for sustainable development in Nepal
- to conduct research into the therapeutic efficacy of Ayurvedic remedies and the medicinal plants available in the country
- to document the healing practices and medicinal plants used by indigenous and local communities and to assess their efficacy.

Activities: A cultivation programme for medicinal plants is being initiated and promoted. Courses for foreign universities are being set up. A database has been created to be used in agricultural, ecological, economic, medical and pharmaceutical research, and research results are being published in brochures and scientific papers.

Geographic interest: Himalayan regions of Nepal.

Database: A database is available with information on medicinal plants in Nepal.

Information/resources: Brochures are published.

Funding: Funding of the institute is through individual contributions and a project fund.

Contact persons: Prof. Dr. L. M. Singh and Mr. R. H. Subedi.

Address: Himalayan Ayurveda Research Institute, P.O. Box 2931, New Plaza, Kathmandu, Nepal. Tel. (+977) 1 / 228625, Fax (+977) 1 / 244617.

Department of Biology, Muscat

Oman

Status: The Department of Biology belongs to Sultan Qaboos University.

Objectives:

- to compile an inventory of medicinal plants used in the Sultanate of Oman
- the describe the uses of medicinal plants by local people
- to study chemical aspects of medicinal plants.

Activities: See objectives. Chemical analyses and laboratory research are also carried out by research laboratories and institutions abroad. In addition to medicinal plants, research is done on plants used in cosmetics and on endangered species.

Geographic interest: Oman and Arabian Peninsula.

Database: The department holds a database of the Sultan Qaboos University Hospital with information on the identification of plants used by patients and livestock poisoning.

Information/resources: No information.

Funding: University funds.

Contact person: Shahina A. Ghazanfar.

Address: Department of Biology, Sultan Qaboos University, P.O. Box 36, Al-Khod 123, Muscat, Sultanate of Oman. Tel.: (+968) 515447 or 513263, Fax: (+968) 513263, e-mail: martinf@squ.edu.

Belour Advisory and Social Development Organisation (BASDO)

Pakistan

Status: Non-governmental organization, registered under the Social Welfare Act and member of IUCN. Founded in 1989, it has currently about 15 members.

Objectives:

- to promote public awareness in the conservation of nature and the protection of natural resources
- to preserve the cultural heritage.

Activities: Special data are collected on the natural ressources of forests, including medicinal plants. The artificial cultivation of critically endangered plant species of medicinal value will be carried out.

Geographic interest: Northern areas of Pakistan.

Database: No computerized database.

Information/resources: A newsletter is published.

Funding: Through donations and membership fees.

Contact person: Ghulam Rasool (general secretary).

Address: Belour Advisory and Social Development Organisation (BASDO), Northern Areas, Domial Road, P.O. Box 501, Gilgit, Pakistan. Tel.: (+92) 572 / 2603, Fax: (+92) 572 / 2779.

Philippines

Indigenous Community Services

Status: *Indigenous Comunity Services, Inc.*, is a non-governmental company with a staff of about 25. The company was founded in 1984 by Jose N. Bangao.

Objective:

- to implement programmes and projects to raise the living conditions of the indigenous cultural communities of Northern Philippines.

Activities: The present work is concentrated on the identification, collection and propagation of all known wild medicinal and pesticidal plants in two selected areas. This includes the establishment of a nursery and the documentation of the names, uses and propagation techniques of these medicinal and pesticidal plants.

Geographic interest: Benguet Province and Mountain Province in Northern Luzon, Philippines.

Database: None.

Information/resources: None.

Funding: Funds are received from various funding agencies and donors.

Contact person: Jose N. Bangao.

Address: Indigenous Community Services, Inc., P.O. Box 665, 2600 Baguio City, Philippines.

Ceylon Institute of Scientific and Industrial Research (CISIR)

Status: Founded in 1955 by the Government of Sri Lanka, it now has a semi-governmental status. The institute comprises approximately 40 researchers, with two of them working on medicinal plants. CISIR is the national focal point of the Asia and Pacific Information Network on Medicinal and Aromatic Plants (APINMAP).

Objectives:
- to conduct phytochemical, pharmacological and analytical studies on medicinal plants
- to prepared value-added products from medicinal plants in pilot studies
- to conduct agronomical studies and to promote the conservation of medicinal plants.

Activities: *Ruellia tuborosa, Alpinia calcarata, Piper longum* and *Kaempheria galanga* are subject of phytochemical studies. An investigation is made on intercropping coconut with seven selected medicinal plants. Anti-inflammatory drugs used in Ayurveda are evaluated and standardizations are recommended. Value-added products such as burn creams, face creams, shampoos, sun protection creams from *Aloe vera* and other medicinal plants are developed for the local market and for export. Extracts are prepared from medicinal plants for export and standardizations are made for Ayurvedic preparations.

Geographic interest: Sri Lanka.

Database: A database has been established within the framework of APINMAP.

Information/resources: Papers in scientific journals, the *IUPAC Congress on Natural Products* and the *Asian Symposia on Medicinal and Aromatic Plants.*

Funding: Funds are received from the Government of Sri Lanka, and some research projects are supported by international organizations.

Contact person: Dr. Lakshmi S. R. Arambewela.

Address: Ceylon Institute of Scientific and Industrial Research (CISIR), 363, Bauddhaloka Mawatha, P.O. Box 787, Colombo 07, Sri Lanka. - Tel.: (+94) 1 / 693807 or 693808, Fax: (+94) 1 / 686567, e-mail: isra@cisir.ac.lk.

Sri Lanka

Department of Chemistry, Nugegoda

Status: Institute of the University of Sri Jayewardenepura. The working group on medicinal plants was initiated by Prof. Tuley de Silva in about 1980.

Objective:
- to study medicinal plants ethnopharmacognostically.

Activities: An attempt is made to study and correlate the chemistry of medicinal plants through plausible bioactivity studies with ethnomedical usages and ethnopharmacology. These studies help in the development of meaningful standards for traditional complex drugs, and in the development of modern forms of traditional drugs. Searches are made for plant immunomodulators. Special emphasis is put on threatened species.

Geographic interest: Sri Lanka.

Database: None.

Information/resources: Articles in various magazines.

Funding: In addition to university funds, there is support from industry and NARESA.

Contact person: Prof. A. M. Abeysekera.

Address: Department of Chemistry, University of Sri Jayewardenepura, Nugegoda, Sri Lanka. Tel.: (+94) 1 / 854206, Fax: (+94) 1 / 852604, e-mail: ajitabey@sjp.ac.lk.

Vietnam

Centre for Research and Development of Ethnomedicinal Plants (CREDEP)

Status: Non-governmental institution founded in 1993 by Prof. Dr. Tran Cong Khanh. At present it has a staff of 20.

Objectives:
- to explore and study the fundamentals of, and experiment with, the productive development of the ethnomedicinal plants and ingredients of the national minorities in Vietnam
- to maintain and develop traditional knowledge for the prevention and cure of diseases among the people
- to plan the conservation, management and development of the medicinal resources.

Activities: There are four current projects: an assessment is made of the potential medicinal value of plants in the Cuc Phuong National Park, for their sustainable utilization and conservation; an ethnobotanical screening programme of the San Chay minority in North Vietnam is carried out, and also an investigation for the protection of genetic diversity of medicinal plants in Phu Luong District, Bac Thai Province; traditional prescriptions for anti-goitre are surveyed.

Geographic interest: Vietnam.

Database: None.

Information/resources: Regular seminars are held.

Funding: No information available.

Contact person: Prof. Dr. Tran Cong Khanh (director).

Address: Centre for Research and Development of Ethnomedicinal Plants (CREDEP), 9, Vu Huu Loi St., Hai Ba Trung Dist., Hanoi, Vietnam. Tel./Fax: (+84) 4 / 8269043.

Australia and Pacific Islands

Australia

The Organic Herb Growers of Australia, Inc.

Status: Incorporated body founded in 1987 by Howard Rubin with approximately 500 members.

Objective:
- to promote and foster the development of an Australian organic herb growing industry.

Activities: Herbs are grown organically and research experiments are carried out with crops. Plants covered are medicinal plants, culinary herbs, and herbs used in cosmetics.

Geographic interest: Australia.

Database: On membership only.

Information/resources: The bi-monthly journal *Herb Grower* is published and bi-monthly meetings are held.

Funding: Membership fees.

Address: Organic Herb Growers of Australia Inc., P.O. Box 6171, South Lismore 2480, Australia. Fax: (+61) 66 / 291057.

New Zealand

Biodiversity, Crops & Food Research Unit

Status: This research unit is part of the Invermay Agricultural Research Centre, which became independent from the Ministry of Agriculture and Fisheries in 1992. The research unit is liked by agreement with the *Fundación Amigos de la Naturaleza* (Bolivia).

Objective:
- to research and develop crops and cultivation techniques to improve New Zealand's agricultural capability while conserving the base for sustainable development.

Activities: Research is done on plant extracts. Bioassays are carried out in order to find out the pharmaceutical effectiveness of certain medicinal plants. Experiments are done on cultivation and biodiversity activities including plant screening, ethnobiology and conservation.

Geographic interest: New Zealand, with some activities in South America.

Database: For personal use only.

Information/resources: The *Lesser Known Plants Newsletter* is published by the group. Broadsheets are used in conservation programmes and papers are published in various journals.

Funding: Funds are received from the government and from private enterprises.

Contact person: Stephan Halloy.

Address: Biodiversity, Crop & Food Research Unit, Invermay Agricultural Research Centre,P.O. Box 50034, Mosgiel, New Zealand. Tel.: (+64) 3 / 4893-809, Fax: (+64) 3 / 4893-739.

Chemistry Department of the University of Papua New Guinea

Papua New Guinea

Status: University institute. There is an affiliated private company, Papua New Guinea Natural Products Pty Ltd., which exports natural products including medicinal plants from Papua New Guinea.

Objective:
- to identify medicinal plants of Papua New Guinea and to evaluate them.

Activities: Medicinal and other economically important plants are identified and their chemical properties studied in the laboratory. Studies are focussed on plants used by local communities against ashma, TB and diabetes and other tropical disorders.

Geographic interest: Papua New Guinea.

Database: No information.

Information/resources: No information.

Funding: Government funds for the university department.

Contact person: Dr. Topul Rali.

Address: Chemistry Department, University of Papua New Guinea, P.O. Box 320, Papua New Guinea.

Wau Ecology Institute

Papua New Guinea

Status: Non-governmental institute, founded in 1972.

Objectives:
- to carry out research on the nature of Papua New Guinea
- to carry out education and public awareness programmes for the conservation of nature.

Activities: Wau Ecology Institute has had an ongoing Medicinal Plants Programme since 1984. A handbook on the medicinal plants of Papua New Guinea is being prepared.

Geographic interest: Papua New Guinea.

Database: None.

Information/resources: Several articles on medicinal plants have been published in international journals, and a handbook on the medicinal plants of Papua New Guinea is being prepared. The first volume dealing with the medicinal plants of Morobe was published five years ago and the volume covering New Guinea is almost finished.

Funding: No information available.

Contact person: Harry Sakulas (director).

Address: Wau Ecology Institute, P.O. Box 77, Wau, Papua New Guinea. Tel.: (+675) 44-6341, Fax: (+675) 44-6381, e-mail: peg:wei.

S. Pacific: Samoa Tonga

Seacology Foundation

Status: Non-governmental, non-profit organization founded in 1988 by Dr. Paul Alan Cox of Brigham Young University.

Objective:
- to preserve the rainforest of the South Pacific, in particular in Samoa and Tonga.

Activities: The foundation supports the building of schools, hospitals, installing water supplies etc. In exchange for these public works, the village councils sign covenants which make it possible to put rainforest acreage into nature reserves with government protection from logging. In collaboration with native Samoan plant healers, medicinal plants are surveyed. Testing their biological activity is done together with the *NCI Laboratory of Drug Discovery Research* and Development and the *NCI Natural Products Branch*. The Anti-AIDS activity of the medicinal plant *Homolanthus nutans* has already been identified and is the subject of further studies.

Geographic interest: Samoa Islands (Western and American Samoa), Tonga.

Database: An address database for mailing newsletters and brochures has been established.

Information/resources: A newsletter is published bi-annually and various leaflets on the objectives and activities of the foundation are available. A video on the conservation of the Samoan rainforest has been produced.

Funding: Personal and corporate donations. There is a capacity to fund the projects of other initiatives and organizations.

Contact person: Lorraine R. Clark (executive associate director).

Address: The Seacology Foundation, P.O. Box 4000, Springville, Utah 84663, U.S.A. Tel.: (+1) 801 / 489-1728, Fax: (+1) 801 / 489-1700, e-mail: lorrainec@murpock.com.

University of South Pacific

S. Pacific

Status: At the University of South Pacific, there are some 10 scientists with medicinal plants interests.

Objectives:
- to identify useful medicinal plants
- to integrate medicinal plants into the formal health care system
- to promote conservation programmes
- to train students on medicinal plants
- to take care of policy development for equitable bioprospecting
- to isolate biological active compounds
- to gather ethnobotanical information.

Activities: There is a rapid appraisal of medicinal plants used by rural people. The information gathered is shared by different parties and a conservation strategy is being developed. Simple activity tests are made by the university itself, otherwise joint programmes are carried out with pharmaceutical companies. Biologically active compounds are isolated and structures are elucidated by the Chemistry Department.

Geographic interest: South Pacific (12 countries).

Database: A database with ethnobotanical information has been established.

Information/resources: Papers in scientific journals.

Funding: Projects are funded by university sources and external funds.

Contact person: Bill Aalbersberg.

Address: University of the South Pacific, Suva, Fiji. Tel.: (+679) 313900, Fax: (+679) 302548. e-mail: Aalbersberg@usp.ac.fj.

Europe

Bulgaria

Institute of Botany, Sofia

Status: The institute, with a staff of approximately 12, was founded in 1965 by Acad. D. Jordanov. It belongs to the Bulgarian Academy of Sciences.

Objectives:

- to study the biology of propagation
- to study the chemistry of biological active substances
- to study the ecology of wild medicinal and aromatic plants
- to make recommendations for the preservation and recovery of medicinal and aromatic plants.

Activities: Two projects are being run at present: one is a biological and phytochemical study of protected valuable medicinal and aromatic plants in Bulgaria, the other an investigation of resources of rare medicinal plants in Bulgaria. Most of the medicinal plants dealt with belong to the families Rutaceae, Asteraceae, and Rosaceae.

Geographic interest: Bulgaria.

Information/resources: The journal *Phytologia Balcanica* (Fitologija Bulgaria) is published by the institute. National conferences on botany are organized.

Funding: The main funding comes from the *National Foundation of Scientific Research* and the *Ministry of the Environment*.

Contact persons: Ljuba Nikolova Evstatieva and Antonina Asenova Vitkova.

Address: Institute of Botany, Bulgarian Academy of Sciences, Sofia 1113, Bulgaria. Tel. (+359) 2 / 713-37-67.

Bulgaria

Ministry of Environment, Bulgaria

Status: Government agency.

Objectives:

- to create legislation on the conservation and harvest of medicinal plants
- to implement the regulations and devise a controlling system.

Activities: The ministry is at present involved in a study of the status of endangered medicinal plants. Laws and regulations for collecting medicinal plants are being formulated. Links are made with ethnomedicine, pharmaceutical industry, processing industry and cosmetic industry.

Geographic interest: Bulgaria.

Database: Information on the status and utilization of medicinal plants is available in an electronic database.

Information/resources: Seminars and workshops are held and leaflets and other printed materials are produced.

Funding: Funds are available through the regular government budget and environmental funds. The ministry is able to initiate and fund projects of other groups and organizations.

Contact person: Mrs. Rayna Hardalova.

Address: Ministry of Environment, 67 W. Gladstone str., 1000 Sofia, Bulgaria. Tel. (+359) 2 / 876151 (or 661494), Fax (+359) 2 / 832279 (or 521634).

Institute of Forestry and Nature Conservation

Estonia

Status: It is a government institute, belonging to the Ministry of Environment.

Objectives:
- to investigate and protect rare and endangered plant species of Estonia.

Activities: Programmes are carried out for the protection of endangered plants, including medicinal plants.

Geographic interest: Estonia.

Database: None.

Contact person: Ülle Kukk.

Address: Institute of Forestry and Nature Conservation, Röömu tu 2, Tartu EE 2400, Estonia. Tel.: (+372) 7 / 436707, Fax: (+372) 7 / 436375, e-mail: Lku@Lkuk.tartu.ee.

Pharmaceutical Institute of Tartu University

Estonia
Latvia
Lithuania

Status: University Institute.

Objectives:

- to carry out studies on medicinal plants
- to cultivate medicinal plants
- to teach pharmacognosy.

Activities: A new garden for medicinal plants was established in 1993. Laboratory studies include the analyses of chemical compounds and physiological parameters of medicinal plants. About 90 species in 30 genera are studied.

Geographic interest: The Baltic States Estonia, Latvia and Lituania. Material received from Great Britain and Canada is also studied.

Database: A database of chemical compounds of medicinal plants is being developed.

Information/resources: The journal *Eesti Rohuteadlane* is published by the institute. Annual meetings are held at the institute.

Funding: Project funds are made available by the university. Projects of other groups cannot be funded.

Contact person: Prof. Dr. Elmar Arak.

Address: Pharmazeutisches Institut, Universität Tartu, Jakobistr. 2, 2400 Tartu, Estonia. Tel. (+372) 7 / 465-281, Fax (+372) 7 / 465-440.

Germany

Institut für Pflanzengenetik und Kulturpflanzenforschung (IPK)

Status: Government institute founded in 1992. Successor of the *Institut für Genetik und Kulturpflanzenforschung* of the former German Democratic Republic. The institute, with a total staff of approximately 385 (128 of these scientists), has divisions for taxonomy, chromosomal analysis and cytogenetics, molecular genetics, molecular cell biology, and genebank.

Objectives:

- to collect, evaluate, characterize, preserve and distribute plant germplasm
- to study the evolution of crop plants.

Activities: Comparative studies on cultivated plants and their wild relatives. A three-year project on the diversity of coriander (*Coriandrum sativa* L.) is ongoing. *Ex situ* protection of genetic resources. The genebank contains 269 species of medicinal and aromatic plants.

Geographic interest: Mainly Europe.

Database: None relevant for medicinal plants.

Information/resources: An *Index Seminum Gaterslebensis* is published every two years.

Funding: German government funds.

Contact person: Dipl. Ing.-agr. Axel Diederichsen.

Address: Institut für Pflanzengenetik und Kulturpflanzenforschung - Genbank - Corrensstr. 3, 06466 Gatersleben, Germany. Tel.: (+90) 39482 / 5280, Fax: (+90) 39482 / 5155.

Mediterranean Agronomic Institute of Chania

Greece

Status: Non-governmental institute, a sub-institution of CIHEAM. About 5 people have been working on medicinal plants since 1986.

Objectives:
- to offer a training programme on applied biological sciences leading to a *Specialised Post-University Diploma* and *Master of Science degree.*
- to carry out research in plant production and agricultural systems.

Activities: The institute is running a project on identification, preservation, adaptation and cultivation of selected aromatic and medicinal plants suitable for marginal lands of the Mediterranean region. A model of technical and economic optimisation of specialist minor crops is being developed. An inventory of the uses of aromatic and medicinal plants of Crete is being prepared.

Geographic interest: Greece, in particular Crete, and to some extent also other Mediterranean areas.

Database: A computerized database on the native plant species of Crete has been established.

Information/resources: Regular seminars and workshops.

Funding: Institute funds and projects supported by the European Union (EU).

Contact persons: Alkinoos Nikolaidis (director), Melpo Skoula (researcher), and Christina Fourmaki (researcher).

Address: Mediterranean Agronomic Institute of Chania (MAICH), Alsylion Agrokepion, 73100 Chania, Greece. Tel.: (+30) 821 / 81151-3, Fax: (+30) 821 / 81154, e-mail: melpo(at)@zorbas.maich.gr.

Hungary

Medicine Institute of Pharmacognosy at Semmelweis University

Status: A group of about 10 people around Prof. Dr. Petri at the Medicine Institute of Pharmacognosy is working on medicinal plants.

Objectives:
- to teach undergraduate students and postgraduate pharmacists basic knowledge on medicinal plants (pharmacognosy, phytochemistry, biotechnology)
- to investigate medicinal plants and plants containing essential oils and polyphenols.

Activities: Activities are focussed on developing new plant products based on ethnobotanical surveys and clinical experiments. New analytical methods are developed and the efficacy of related legislation is examined.

Geographic interest: Hungary.

Database: None.

Information/resources: Not known.

Funding: Funding is through OTKA, the Hungarian Scientific Research Foundation.

Contact person: Prof. Dr. Gizela Petri.

Address: Medicine Institute of Pharmacognosy, Semmelweis University, Budapest, Hungary. Tel./Fax: (+36) 1 / 1138-608.

Hungary

Research Institute for Medicinal Plants, Budapest

Status: The Research Institute for Medicinal Plants (RIMP) is a non-governmental institute, founded in 1915. It has a regular membership of approximately 110.

Objectives:
- to promote research on and technological development of medicinal plant production
- to develop manufacturing techniques of products from medicinal plants
- to produce seeds, medicinal plants, herbal medicines
- to offer training capacities.

Activities: See objectives.

Geographic interest: Hungary, in particular the surroundings of Budapest.

Database: Much of the information obtained is stored in computerized databases.

Information: The *Joumal of Planar Chromatography - Modem TLC* is being published by the institute. A newsletter *Joumal of Medicinal and Aromatic Plants* is being developed. Congresses, seminars and workshops are regularly held in Hungary and abroad.

Funding: The institute is able to fund projects which contribute to the overall objectives of the institute.

Contact person: Prof. Dr. Sz. Nyiredy.

Address: Research Institute for Medicinal Plants, P.O. Box 11, 2011 Budakalész, Hungary. Tel. (+36) 26 / 340203, Fax (+36) 26 / 340426.

Istituto Sperimentale per l'Assestamento Forestale e par l'Alpicoltura (ISAFA)

Italy

Status: Government institute operating since 1973.

Objectives:

- to study the cultivation of some medicinal and aromatic plants
- to create new varieties of medicinal and aromatic plants with improved characteristics.

Activities: Agrotechnical and genetic aspects of several species are studied and insecticidal and pesticidal plants are included.

Geographic interest: Italy.

Database: A computerized database for information on aromatic, medicinal and insecticidal plants has been established.

Information/resources: Scientific papers and an international congress in 1994.

Funding: The work of the institute is funded by the Ministry of Agriculture.

Contact person: Alessandro Bezzi.

Address: Istituto Sperimentale per l'Assestamento Forestale e par l'Alpicoltura, 38050 Villazzano (Trento), Piazze Nicolini 6, Italy. Tel.: (+39) 461 / 924248, Fax (+39) 461 / 914651, e-mail: ISAFA@tqs.it.

Poland

Research Institute of Medicinal Plants, Poznan

Status: Government institution founded by the Polish Government in 1947.

Objectives:

- to carry out research in botany, in plant breeding and agriculture, in phytochemistry, in pharmacology, and in analysis and control
- to produce natural pharmaceutical products for treatment and prophylaxis.

Activities: The institute focusses its activity on scientific and technological subjects connected with raw materials, herbal products and preparations. Breeding and re-introduction of endangered species is carried out.

Geographic interest: Poland (plus Europe and Asia.).

Database: A literature database was established.

Information/resources: The journal *Herba Polonica* and the *Index Seminum* has been published.

Funding: Funds are received from the *State Committee for Scientific Research* and from contracts with the herbal industry.

Contact person: Violetta Sliwinska.

Address: Research Institute of Medicinal Plants (Instytut Roslin i Przetworów Zielarskich), ul. Libelta 27, 61-707 Poznan, Poland. Tel.: (+48) 61 / 524-003, Fax: (+48) 61 / 527-463.

Spain

Grupo de Trabajo, Jaca

Status: Research centre belonging to the government.

Objectives:

- to carry out ecological research.

Activities: Present work includes a survey of medicinal plants and their popular uses in the Pyrenees.

Geographic interest: Spain, in particular the northeast and the Pyrenees.

Database: A database on herbarium material is available.

Information/resources: Various articles and two books.

Funding: Government.

Contact person: Luis Villar Pérez.

Address: Grupo de Trabajo, Jaca, Instituto Pirenaico de Ecología, Avda. Regto. Galicia s/n., Aptdo. 64, 22700 Jaca, Huesca, Spain.

Real Jardin Botanico de Madrid

Spain

Status: Government botanical garden. Work on medicinal plants has been carried out since 1991.

Objectives:
- to further the public interest in plants
- to carry out investigations on economically important plants.

Activities: A research programme is carried out on ethnobotany in Spain and on the use of plants in folk medicine.

Geographic interest: Spain.

Database: None.

Information/resources: Seminars and workshops are held regularly and workshop papers are published.

Funding: Government.

Contact persons: Emilio Blanco, Ramon Morales and Manuel Macía.

Address: Real Jardin Botanico de Madrid, Pza. de Murillo 2, 28014 Madrid, Spain.

Division of Pharmacognosy, Uppsala

Sweden

Status: Institute of Uppsala University.

Objectives:
- to offer an education programme in the subject of pharmacognosy at

undergraduate level

- to take responsibility for graduate studies to Ph.D. in the subject of pharmacognosy
- to develop and implement research programmes.

Activities: Current projects include structure-activity studies of compounds isolated from medicinal plants with anti-inflammatory activity. Also biologically active peptides are studied.

Geographic interest: Sweden.

Database: None.

Information/resources: Articles in scientific journals.

Funding: Funds are received from the University of Uppsala and from the Research Council of Sweden.

Contact person: Lars Bohlin.

Address: Division of Pharmacognosy, Husargatan 3, D7, plan 5, Uppsala (visiting address), Biomedicum, Box 579, S-75123 Uppsala, Sweden (postal address). Tel.: (+46) 18 / 174000, Fax: (+46) 18 / 509101, e-mail: lars-bohlin@pharmacog.uu.se.

Turkey

Department of Pharmaceutical Botany, Istanbul University

Status: A permanent working group of approximately five people at the Department of Pharmaceutical Botany deals with medicinal plants.

Objectives:

- to make scientific identifications of the wild plants which are used especially for food and medicine by local people
- to study traditional knowledge on the usage of plants in health care
- to bridge the gap between folk and modern medicine and to determine the similarities and differences between them
- to determine the factors affecting the habitats of the plants which are used in different ways and to make recommendations for their conservation
- to investigate the usage and vernacular names of economically important plants.

Activities: Field excursions are made to identify plant species, to collect them, and to record vernacular names and ethnomedical uses. Interviews are made with local people. The abundance of some plant species and the factors threatening them are determined. Specimens collected in the field are kept in a herbarium at the Faculty of Pharmacy, and scientific identifications and descriptions are made accordingly.

Geographic interest: Turkey.

Database: Databases are available for the geographic distribution of plant species in Turkey and for the vernacular names of plant species.

Information/resources: The scientific magazine *Journal of the Faculty of Pharmacy of Istanbul University* is published semi-annually. Irregular seminars are held in the department, and *Vegetable Crude Drugs Meetings* are organized together with other Turkish Faculties of Pharmacy at two-year intervals.

Funding: Funding is through the *Scientific and Technical Research Council of Turkey* (TÜBITAK) and research funds of the university.

Contact person: Assoc. Prof. Dr. Kerim Alpinar.

Address: Department of Pharmaceutical Botany, Faculty of Pharmacy, University of Istanbul, 34452 Üniversite, Istanbul, Turkey. Tel.: (+90) 212 / 5140364, Fax: (+90) 212 / 5190812.

Department of Pharmacognosy, Gazi University, Ankara

Turkey

Status: University institute founded in 1982. There are 22 staff.

Objectives:
- to analyse the pharmacology and chemistry of medicinal plants and to study the biological activity of Turkish folk medicines
- to isolate biological active compounds from medicinal plants
- to collect and evaluate folk medicinal information in Turkey and to prepare a folk medicine inventory
- to standardize phytopharmaceuticals.

Activities: Extensive ethnopharmacological field surveys are performed on an annual basis. Research has concentrated on antiulcerogenic, antiinflammatory, antiulcer, antirheumatic, antidiabetic, antihepatotoxic, antibacterial, and antifungal activities. The collected plant material is analysed in the laboratory. Some phytochemical studies on Labiatae are conducted.

Geographic interest: Turkey.

Database: None.

Information/resources: More than 200 papers and reports have been published in scientific journals. Regular national congresses are held.

Funding: Main funds are received from the university and the *Scientific and Technical Research Council of Turkey* (TÜBITAK). Some activities have been supported by foreign organizations such as NATO and the Japanese Ministry of Science and Culture.

Contact persons: Prof. Dr. Ekrem Sezik and Prof. Dr. Erdem Yesilada.

Address: Gazi University, Faculty of Pharmacy, Department of Pharmacognosy, 06330 Hipodrom, Ankara, Turkey. Tel.: (+90) 312 / 2151113 or 2235018, Fax: (+90) 312 / 2210649 or 2224255.

Turkey

Medicinal and Aromatic Plant and Drug Research Centre

Status: The *Medicinal and Aromatic Plant and Drug Research Centre* (TBAM) was formerly known under the name *Medicinal Plant Research Centre* and belongs to Anadolu University at Eskisehir, Turkey. The centre was founded in 1982. The facilities were greatly extended in1986, and at present it has a technical and scientific staff of about 25.

Objectives:
- to conduct pilot studies for the industrial processing and quality control of materials from plants used in pharmaceuticals, foods, perfumes, cosmetics, dyes, etc.
- to contribute to the development of a sustainable use of the plants of Turkey
- to offer training courses on processing and quality control of plant materials for people from the industry
- to evaluate the flora of Turkey.

Activities: Current activities include the establishment of a herbarium (ESSE), which has at present over 12,000 specimens from all over Turkey; excursions for plant screening to various parts of Turkey, processing of medicinal and aromatic plants, bioassays, formulation of pharmaceutical and cosmetic products, development of training techniques, collection of ethnobotanical information. The training courses offered include *Training on Medicinal and Aromatic Plants in Pharmaceutical and related Industries* (TRUMAP) offered annually in September for 25 days.

Geographic interest: Turkey.

Database: Bibliographic database on medicinal and aromatic plants of Turkey.

Information/resources: The institute publishes TABBÜLTENI (Medicinal and Aromatic Plants Bulletin, in Turkish with English abstracts) with 1–2 issues per year, and *TRUMAP Newsletter* with one issue per year. Over 200 papers in scientific journals. A Turkish-Uzbek symposium on the chemistry of natural compounds is held once every two years, alternately in Uzbekistan and Turkey.

Funding: The work of the institute is funded by UNDP and UNIDO, by the Government of Turkey and by funds generated through services to the industry.

Contact person: Prof. Dr. K. Hüsnü Can Baser (director of TBAM and head of the Pharmaceutical Faculty).

Address: Medicinal and Aromatic Plant and Drug Research Centre, Pharmaceutical Faculty, Anadolu University, 26470 Eskisehir, Turkey. Tel. (+90) 222 / 335-2952, Fax (+90) 222 / 335-0127, e-mail: tbam@vm.baum.anadolu.edu.tr.

The National Institute of Medical Herbalists

United Kingdom

Status: The National Institute of Medical Herbalists was established in 1864 and is the oldest body representing practitioners of herbal medicine in the world. It is a non-governmental organization with over 300 members that have undergone a rigorous four year training and adhere to a strict professional code of ethics.

Objectives:
- to consult herbal practitioners
- to ensure quality standards among medical herbalists
- to strengthen the position of medical herbalists
- to provide the public with addresses of qualified medical herbalists.

Activities: Activities include the training of medical herbalists and the promotion for the improvement of the legislative framework for herbal medicine. A current research project involves medical outcome studies on patients with specific conditions undergoing treatment by medical herbalists.

Geographic interest: United Kingdom.

Database: Computerized address base of practitioners of herbal medicine in U.K.

Information/resources: The journal *European Journal of Herbal Medicine* is published three times a year. Regular meetings and congresses are held for practitioners.

Funding: Membership fees and funding from various bodies for research projects.

Contact person: Alison M. Denham.

Address: The National Institute of Medical Herbalists, 56 Longbrook Street, Exeter EX4 6AH, United Kingdom. Tel.: (+44) 1392 / 426022, Fax: (+44) 1392 / 498963.

United Kingdom

Scottish Agricultural College, Auchincruive

Status: University institute which hosts an „Aromatic and Medicinal Plant Group".

Objectives:
- to study medicinal and aromatic plants and volatile oil crops.

Activities: Activities with medicinal plants include surveys for biological activity. For example, antibacterial, antimycotic and antioxidant activities are studied.

Geographic interest: Great Britain and collaboration with other countries, including Japan, Finland, Israel and other E.U. countries.

Database: A database for assistance in the production of medicinal herbs is available.

Information/resources: Many articles in scientific journals.

Funding: Private pharmaceutical firms and Government funds.

Contact person: Dr. Katerina Pavla Svoboda.

Address: Scottish Agricultural College, Watson Peat Building, Auchincruive, Ayr KA6 5HW, Scotland, United Kingdom. Tel.: (+44) 1292 / 520331, Fax: (+44) 1292 / 525314, e-mail: K.Svoboda@au.sac.ac.uk.

Information sources

Key Journals and Newsletters

A selection of journals and newsletters is presented here that include contributions on medicinal plant conservation to a variable extent, or that would give the opportunity to publish relevant informations. If inadvertently a journal or newsletter has been missed, please contact the editors so that it can be added to the list in the next edition of the directory.

Advances in Economic Botany

is a journal published irregularly since 1983 by the New York Botanical Garden. It is an interdisciplinary series designed to integrate pure and applied studies. The contents are mainly research papers and symposia dealing with the uses and management of plants.

Editor:	Padoch, C.
Address:	New York Botanical Garden, Scientific Publications Department, Bronx, NY 10458-5126, USA, Fax (+1) 718/220-6504.
ISSN:	0741-8280

Ambio

is an international journal, published eight times a year by the Royal Swedish Academy of Sciences. *Ambio* provides articles on developments and issues in environmental research, policy and related activities, including environmental management, sustainable technology and use of natural resources.

Editor:	Kessler, E.
Address:	P. O. Box 50005, S-10405 Stockholm, Sweden, Fax (+46) 8 / 166251.
ISSN:	0044-7447

Amruth

A quaterly newsletter published by the Foundation for the Revitalization of Local Health Traditions (FRLHT). Point focus of *Amruth* is to disseminate information on medicinal plants conservation efforts.

Medicinal plants issues related to primary health care, economics, politics, history, culture and conservation science are also addressed.

Editor: Thayil, S.
Address: FRLHT, 50, MSH Layout, 2nd Stage, 3rd Main, Anandnagar, Bangalore 560024, India, Fax (+91) 803334167
ISSN: 0971-6793

Apinmap Newsletter

is a newsletter published by the Tropical Forest Medicinal Programme.

Editor: Ir Ervizal Zuhud
Address: Dept. of Forest Resource Conservation, Bogor Agricultural University, Kampus IPB Darmaga, P.O. Box 168, Bogor 16001, Indonesia.

Botanical and Herb Reviews

is a newsletter published quarterly.

Editor: Foster, S.
Address: P.O. Box 1343, Fayetteville, Arkansas 72702, USA.
ISSN: 1047-000X

Bulletin of Medico-Ethno-Botanical Research

is a quarterly journal published by the Central Council for Research in Ayurveda and Siddha. It covers folk medicine, pharmacognosy, and phytochemistry, and examines the correlation between ancient insights and modern scientific thought.

Editor: Pandey, V. N.
Address: CCR in Ayurveda and Siddha, Dharma Bhawan, S-10, Green Park Extn. Market, New Dehli 110 016, India.

Business of Herbs

is a bimonthly journal published since 1983. It provides marketing and production techniques, covers government regulatory issues and research on medicinal herbs, and lists useful resources and news for the small herb business.

Editor: Oliver, P. C. & Oliver, D. L.
Address: Northwind Farm Publications, Rte. 2, P.O. Box 246, Shevlin, MN 56676-9535, USA, (+1) 318/657-2447.
ISSN: 0736-9050

Current Advances in Ecological and Environmental Sciences

(former *Current Advances in Ecological Sciences*) is a monthly abstracts journal which gives listings of titles of ecological papers published throughout the world, classified into 61 main areas. This comprehensive literature searching service is used by biologists, ecologists and environmental scientists. It is also avilable as diskette edition (ISSN 1350-6528) and on online.

Editor: Greener, A.
Address: Oxford Fulfilment Centre, Elsevier Science, PO Box 800, Kidlington, Oxford, OX5 1DX, UK, (+44) 865/843010.
ISSN: 0955-6648

Current Research on Medicinal and Aromatic Plants

is a quarterly abstracts journal published since 1979 by the Central Institute of Medicinal and Aromatic Plants. Former name of the journal was *Central Indian Medicinal Plants Organisation Newsletter.*

Editor: Shri O.P. Virmani
Address: Council of Scientific and Industrial Research, P.O. Box 1, P.O. Ram Sagar Misra Nagar, Lucknow 226016, India.
ISSN: 0253-7125

Drogenreport

is a semiannually journal published since 1988 by the Artemisia e.V., Wissenschaftlich-technischer Informationskreis Artern/Thüringen (i.G.).

Editor: Artemisia e.V.
Address: E. Eichholz, Am Westbahnhof, D-06556 Artern.
ISSN: 0863-1816

Economic Botany

is a quarterly journal published since 1947 by the Society of Economic Botany.

Editor: Kaplan, L.
Address: New York Botanical Garden, Scientific Publications Department, Bronx, NY 10458-5126, USA, Fax (+1) 718/220-6504.
ISSN: 0013-0001

Ethnobotany

is a semiannual journal published since 1989 by the Society of Ethnobotanists. *Ethnobotany* bridges the gap between pure and applied botany by focusing on the uses of plants by people.

Editor: Jain, S. K.
Address: Deep Publications, A-3-27-A DDA Flats, Paschim Vihar, New Dehli 110063, India.
ISSN: 0971-1252

Fitoterapia

is a bimonthly journal published since 1934 by Indena. It covers reviews on study and application of medicinal plants. The articles are in English, French or Italian. English summaries are always given. *Fitoterapia* is also available on online.

Editor: Bonati, A.
Address: IdB Holding, Via Ripamonti, 20141 Milano, Italy, Fax (++39) 2 / 57496290.
ISSN: 0367-326X

Foster's Botanical and Herb Review

is an abstracts journal published quarterly.

Editor: Steven Foster
Address: Steven Foster, P.O. Box 1343, Fayetteville, AR 72702, USA.

G-15 Gene Banks for Medicinal & Aromatic Plants Newsletter

is a semiannually newsletter published since 1992 by the Ministry of Science & Technology. It aims to disseminate information about the scientific conservation and economical utilization aspects of medicinal plants amongst the G-15 nations.

Editor:	Sharma, M. & Natesh, S.
Address:	Department of Biotechnology, Block-2, 6-8th floor, CGO Complex, Lodi Road, New Dehli 110003, India.

Herb, Spice and Medicinal Plant Digest

is a quarterly newsletter published since 1983 by the Department of Plant and Soil Sciences, University Massachusetts. Each issue contains a feature article devoted to some aspect related to the production, processing, and/or marketing of herbs, spices, and medicinal plants. In addition, the current herbal literature is reviewed and profiles related to herbal history are developed.

Editor:	Craker, L. E. & Simon, J. E.
Address:	Department of Plant and Soil Sciences, Stockbridge Hall, University of Massachusetts, Amherst, MA 01003, USA, Fax (+1) 413 / 545-1242.
ISSN:	1048-3160

Herba Polonica

is a quarterly journal published since 1955 by the Research Institute of Medicinal Plants, Poznan. It is cosponsored by the Polish Ministry of Agriculture and Food Economy. Its articles are published in English, German or Polish. Summaries and abstracts are given in English and Russian. *Herba Polonica* is also available on online.

Address:	Instytut Róslin i Przetworów Zielarskich, ul. Libelta 27, 61-707 Poznan, Poland, Fax (+48) 61 / 527462.
ISSN:	0018-0599

Herbalgram

is a quarterly journal published since 1979 by the American Botanical Council and The Herb Research Foundation. It provides following informations on herbs and medicinal plants, both within the USA and internationally: current research aspects, literature reviews, conferences, legal and market update.

Editor:	Blumenthal, M.
Address:	ABC, P.O. Box 201660 Austin, Texas, 78720, Fax (+1) 512 / 331-1924.
ISSN:	0899-5648

Horticultural Abstracts

is a monthly abstracts journal published since 1931 by the Centre for Agriculture and Biosciences International (CABI). For more information on CABI: see Databases.

Address:	CAB International, Library Services Centre, Silwood Park, Buckhorst Rd., Ascot, Berks SL5 7TA, U.K., Fax (+44) 1344 / 872901.
ISSN:	0018-5280

ICMAP Newsletter

is a biannually newsletter published since 1995 by the International Council for Medicinal and Aromatic Plants. ICMAP Newsletter provides information of international importance and reviews of meetings, workshops and publications. Additionally it is intended to publish country reports which give special attention to production, development programmes, scientific activity and other relevant facts of one country.

Address:	ICMAP Secretariat, c/o IUBS, 51 Boulevard de Montmorency, 75016 Paris, France.

IMP News

is a newsletter published by the International Medicinal Plants Network.

Address:	IMPN, IRDC, South Asia Regional Office, 17, Jor Bagh, New Delhi 110003, India.

Inmedplan. The Indian Medicinal Plant Distributed Databases Network

is a newsletter published since 1994 by the Foundation for the Revitalization of Local Health Traditions (FRLHT). It covers the development within this databases network, and highlights related news both in India and abroad.

Address: FRLHT, 50, MSH Layout, 2nd Stage, 3rd Main, Anandnagar, Bangalore 560024, India, Fax (+91) 803334167

International Pharmaceutical Abstracts

is a semiannually abstracts journal published since 1964 by the American Society of Hospital Pharmacists. It is scanning the world's literature of pharmacy, covering approximately 800 pharmaceutical, medical and health care publications. The *International Pharmaceutical Abstracts* are also available on online and on CD-ROM

Editor: Tousignaut, D. R.
Address: ASHP / c/o Jean Rogers, Mkt. Svcs., 7272 Wisconsin Ave, Bethesda, MD 20814, USA, Fax (+1) 302 / 657-1641.
ISSN: 0020-8264

Journal of Applied Botany

(former *Angewandte Botanik*) is published since 1919 by the Vereinigung für Angewandte Botanik. Each year three double issues are published.

Editor: Jäger, H. J.
Address: Dr. Herwig Koch, Grisebachstraße 6, D-37077 Göttingen, Germany.
ISSN: 0066-1759

Journal of Ethnobiology

is a semiannually journal published since 1981 by the Society of Ethnobiology. It features articles about the uses of plants and animals by native people worldwide, both prehistorically and historically. The abstracts are given in English, French and Spanish.

Editor: Pearsall, D.
Address: Brien A. Meilleur, Missouri Botanical Garden, Center for Plant Conservation, P.O. Box 299, St. Louis MO 63166.
ISSN: 0278-0771

Journal of Ethnopharmacology

is an interdisciplinary journal published monthly since 1979. It is devoted to bioscientific research on indigenous drugs. The *Journal of Ethnopharmacology* publishes original articles concerned with the observation and experimental investigation of the biological activity of plant and animal substances used in traditional medicine of past and present cultures. It also provides abstracts of current literature screened from more than 100 journals.

Editor:	Rivier, L. & Soejarto, D. D.
Address:	Elsevier Science Ireland Ltd., P.O. Box 85, Limerick, Ireland, Fax (+353) 61 / 472144.
ISSN:	0378-8741

Journal of Herbs, Spices and Medicinal Plants

is a quarterly journal published since 1991. It features original articles and short reviews associated with the production and development of herbs, spices, and medicinal plants. The provided informations are related to such areas as physiology, breeding, productivity, commercial applications, and marketing.

Editor:	Craker, L. E.
Address:	The Haworth Press Inc., 10 Alice Street, Binghamtoon, NY 13904-1580, USA, Fax (+1) 607 / 722-1424.
ISSN:	1049-6475

Journal of Medicinal and Aromatic Plants

(former *Herba Hungarica)* is a journal published since 1962 by the Hungarian Research Institute of Medicinal and Aromatic Plants. Each year are appearing three volumes. The articles are written in English language.

Editor:	Bernath, J.
Address:	Gyogynoveny Kutato Intezet, P.O.B. 11, 2011 Budakalasz, Hungary.
ISSN:	0018-0580

Journal of Natural Products

(former *Llodya*) is a monthly trade journal published since 1931 by the American Society of Pharmacognosy and The Lloyd Library and Museum. It covers all aspects of natural product research, from chemistry of naturally occuring compounds to biology of the living systems from which they are obtained. The *Journal of Natural Products* is also available on online.

Editor:	Kinghorn, A. D.
Address:	The American Society of Pharmacognosy, c/o D. J. Slatkin, Chicago Coll. of Pharmacy, 555 31st Street, Downers Grove, Illinois 60515, USA, Fax (+1) 708 / 9716097.
ISSN:	0163-3864

Medicinal and Aromatic Plants Abstracts

(former *Bulletin of Indian Raw Materials and their Utilization*) is a bimonthly abstracts journal published since 1979 by the Council of Scientific and Industrial Research. It reports current world literature on medicinal and aromatic plants, covering about 600 journals published in 22 languages from 55 countries of the world. It includes patents and papers presented at the national and international seminars and symposia in the field. It includes, in particular, reviews of Chinese literature. Each issue contains approximately 700 abstracts. The abstracts are available on online.

Editor:	Jain, H. C.
Address:	Dr. K. S. Krishnan Marg, Senior Sales and Distr. Officer, Publications and Information Directorate, New Dehli 110 012, India, Fax: (+91) 11 / 5731353.
ISSN:	0250-4367

Medicinal Plant Conservation

is an annually newsletter published since 1995 by the IUCN/SSC Medicinal Plant Specialist Group (MPSG). In addition to news on the development within the MPSG, organizations and projects are presented.

Editor:	Cunningham, A. B. & Schippmann, U.
Address:	MPSG, Bundesamt für Naturschutz, Konstantinstraße 110, D-53177 Bonn, Germany.
ISSN:	1430-953X

Medicinal Plants Conservation

is a newsletter published by the Centre for Environmental Research.

Address: CER, Third Science Building, University of Rajshahi, Rajshahi 6205, Bangladesh.

MFP News

is a quarterly newsletter published since 1991 by the Society of the Centre of Minor Forest Products. Purpose of the publication is to strengthen capabilities of state forest departments, offer assistance to all user groups and render help in improving the socio-economic condition of the forest and village dwellers including tribals.

Editor: Agarwal, V. S.
Address: HIG-2, No.8, Indirapuram, Gen. Mahadev Singh Road, P.O. Majra, Dehra Dun 248 171, India.

NANMAP. A Bimonthly Newsletter of the Asian Network on Medicinal and Aromatic Plants

(fromerly: *BANMAP*) is a bimonthly newsletter published since 1993 by the Asian Network on Medicinal and Aromatic Plants (ANMAP).

Editor: Chomchalow, N.
Address: ANMAP Secretariat, FAO Regional Office for Asia and the Pacific, Maliwan Mansion, Phrai Atit Road, Bangkok 10200, Thailand, Fax (+662) 280 / 0445.

NAPRECA Newsletter

is published by the Natural Products Research Network for Eastern and Central Africa.

Editor: Nkunya, M. H. H.
Address: Chemistry Departement, University of Dar es Salaam, P.O. Box 35061, Dar es Salaam, Tanzania.
ISSN: 1022-3177

Nature and Resources

(former *Nature & Resources and Man and Biosphere Program. Bulletin*) is a quarterly journal published since 1958 by the UNESCO. It contains international news about research on environment, resources, and conservation of nature. Emphasis is given to current symposia and conferences. *Nature and Resources* is edited in English, French or Spanish.

Editor: Lasserre, P. & Hadley, M.
Address: Parthenon Publishing Group, Casterton Hall, Carnforth, Lancs LA6 2LA, U.K.
ISSN: 0547-9665

Non Wood News

is an annual journal published since 1994 by the Non-Wood Products and Energy Branch (FOPN), FAO. Besides international news, it provides comprehensive chapters on products and market and on regional aspects of commercialisation and sustainable use of non-timber forest products. Additionally, *Non Wood News* contains a calendar of recent and forthcoming events, and a review of current publications.

Editor: Chandrasekharan, C. & Léger, C.
Address: Non-Wood Products and Energy Branch (FOPN), FAO, Viale delle Terme de Caracalla, Roma, Italy.
ISSN: 1020-3435

People and Plants Handbook

is a handbook edited in a serial of journal issues by the People and Plant Intiative of UNESCO, WWF and Royal Botanic Gardens, Kew. Main objective of the handbook is to present sources for applying ethnobotany to conservation and community development. The first issue, published in 1996, deals with journals and organisations in this field.

Editor: Martin, G. J.
Address: People and Plants Initiative, Division of Ecological Sciences, UNESCO, 7 place de Fontenoy, 75352 Paris Cedex 07 SP, France, Fax (+33) 1 / 40659897.

Plant Talk

is a quarterly journal published since 1995 by the Botanical Information Company Ltd. It covers issues and events in plant conservation worldwide, reviews on Red Data Books, and information on new protected areas.

Editor:	Akeroyd, J. & Synge, H.
Address:	P.O. Box 500, Kingston-upon-Thames, Surrey KT2 5XB, U.K.; or: P.O. Box 65226, Tucson, AZ 85728-5226, USA.
ISSN:	1358-4103

Review of Aromatic and Medicinal Plants

is a bimonthly abstracts journal published since 1995 by the Centre for Agriculture and Biosciences International (CABI). It is aimed at research community working in universities and institutes specialising in aromatic and medicinal plants. It will also appeal to those in the pharmaceutical, cosmetic and perfumery industry and to scientists from a wide range of diciplines including pharmacology, natural products chemistry, horticulture and ethnobotany. For more informations on CABI: see Databases.

Address:	CAB International, Library Services Centre, Silwood Park, Buckhurst Rd., Ascot, Berks SL5 7TA, U.K., Fax (+44) 1344 / 872901.
ISSN:	1356-1421

TRAFFIC Bulletin / TRAFFIC International

is a journal published by TRAFFIC International, which is devoted entirely to wildlife trade issues. It covers all aspects of trade in wild animals, plants and derived products.

Editor:	Thomsen, J. & Lochen, K.
Address:	World Conservation Monitoring Centre, 219c, Huntingdon Road, Cambridge, CB3 0DL, U.K., Fax (+44) 223 / 277237.
ISSN:	0267-4297

TRUMAP Newsletter

is an annually newsletter published by the Medicinal and Aromatic Plant and Drug Research Centre (TBAM).

Address: TBAM, Pharmaceutical Faculty, Anadolu University, 26470 Eskisehir, Turkey.

Washington Insight. Newsletter for Natural Products Scientists

is a quarterly newsletter published since 1988.

Editor: Persinos, G. J.
Address: 11000 Waycroft Way, North Bethesda, MD 20852, USA.
ISSN: 0899-7241

Databases

Many groups listed in the directory have established and are maintaining electronic databases where they process the information they collect. In this section a few databases are reviewed which have a general interest and to which there is a public access.

APINMAP Database

APINMAP database belongs to UNESCO and is managed by the *Asian and Pacific Information Network on Medicinal and Aromatic Plants*. It contains literature references on medicinal plants and spices from the Asian and Pacific regions. Diskettes and print-outs are distributed.

The database is freely available to network members. There are some restrictions for external users.

Addresses: Ms. Alice H. Rillo, APINMAP Coordinator, APINMAP Network Centre, Agricultural Information Bank for Asia, Regional Centre for Graduate Study and Research in Agriculture, College, Laguna 4031, Philippines. Tel.: (+63) 42 / 2380 and 2576. **or:** Prof. K. Manunapichu, Ministry of University Affairs, Si Ayutthya Road, Bangkok 10400, Thailand. Fax: (+66) 2 / 2871443. **or:** Dr. Patricia L. Zara, Philippine Council for Health, Research and Development, Department of Science and Technology, Gen. Santos Ave., Bicutan, Taguig, Metro Manilla, Philippines. Fax: (+63) 2 / 8238942 or 8238937.

CAB International

The *Centre for Agriculture and Biosciences International* (CABI or CAB International) is an international, inter-governmental organization established in 1928. It is owned by its member governments, which currently number 36. One of its main issues is *CAB Abstracts*, one of the leading bibliographic databases which covers agriculture, forestry, aspects of human health, and applied sciences. Over 12,000 serials and many other publications are scanned, and over 160,000 bibliographic records are compiled each year for input to CAB International's main databases. One of the numerous printed products derived from this database is the *Review of Aromatic and Medicinal Plants* (see under Key Journals and Newsletters).

Address (headquarters): CAB International, Wallingford, Oxon OX10 8DE, United Kingdom, Tel.: (+44) 1491 / 832111, Fax: (+44) 1491 / 833508.

North America: 845 North Park Avenue, Tucson, Arizona 85719, U.S.A. (Tel.: (+1) 800 / 528-4841 or (+) 602 / 621-7897, Fax (+1) 602 / 621-3816.

Asia: PO Box 11872, 50760 Kuala Lumpur, Malaysia, Tel. (+60) 3 / 255-2922, Fax (+60) 3 / 255-1888.

Carribean: Gordon Street, Curepe, Trinidad and Tobago, Tel. (+1809) 662-4173, Fax (+1809) 663-2859.

Inmedplan (Indian Medicinal Plants Distributed Databases Network)

Inmedplan is a network of nine nodal agencies and several satellite agencies, compiling multi-disciplinary information on plants used for medicine in India. Each nodal agency manages the information in a particular area of data:

- Agrotechnology: Central Institute of Medicinal and Aromatic Plants (CIMAP),
- Bibliography and abstracts: Publication and Information Directorate (PID),
- Botany: Botanical Survey of India,
- Ecology: Dept. of Ecology of the French Institute of Pondicherry,
- Ethnomedicine: Tropical Botanical Garden and Research Insitute (TBGRI),
- Pharmacognosy: Ayurveda Research Institute,
- Pharmacology: Central Drug Research Institute (CDRI),
- Phytochemistry: Regional Research Laboratory (RRL),
- Traditional (indigenous) systems: Centre of Indian Medical Heritage (CIMH)

Objecitve of Inmedplan is to serve the information needs of agriculture, community health, medical research, the pharmaceutical industry and medicinal plants conservation. Enquiries on medicinal plants can be addressed to the Inmedplan Secretariat:

Foundation for Revitalisation of Local Health Traditions (FRLHT)
No. 50, 2nd Stage, 3rd Main, M.S.H. Layout
Anand Nagar, Bangalore 560 024
India
(contact person: Mr. Ravi Chander)
Tel.: (+91) 80 / 3336909
Fax: (+91) 80 / 3334167
e-mail: lnmed@frlht.ernet.in

Inmedplan is liaised with international databases like NAPRALERT, WCMC and others. Currently, Inmedplan is an organised offline distributed network which will provide online access as soon as user demand grows to a viabel level.

NAPRALERT (Natural Products ALERT)

NAPRALERT is a database of the world literature on the chemical constituents and pharmacology of plant, microbial and animal (primarily marine) extracts. In addition, considerable data are contained in NAPRALERT on the chemistry and pharmocology (including human studies) of secondary metabolites of known structure, derived from natural sources. The information-base is currently maintained as an ongoing activity of the Program for Collaborative Research in the Pharmaceutical Sciences (PCRPS) in the College of Pharmacy, University of Illinois at Chicago.

More than 124,000 scientific articles and/or books have been computerized. About 75% of these are from the post-1975 literature. The remaining records are obtained by selective retrospective indexing dating back to 1650. Current issues from approximately 200 scientific journals which have been found to contain information most pertinent to NAPRALERT, based on several years of experience, are monitored. Several abstract services are also scanned, including *Chemical Abstracts, Biological Abstracts, Index Medicus, Medicinal and Aromatic Plant Abstracts, Current Indian Titles*, and *Current Contents-Life Sciences Issue*. The database increases at a rate of approximately 600 articles per month.

The articles contain information on more than 129,000 pure chemical species, more than 48,000 plant, marine, microbial or animal species and more than 1.5 million records which associate these previous record types with biological activity.

Information retrieved ranges from an in-depth three-part profile of any plant species, which would contain three major types of information: ethnomedical, pharmacological and phytochemical. Data retrieval may also focus on specifics, such as chemical constituents, geographic locations or biological activity of any given family, genus or species of organism.

NAPRALERT database is fully accessible, for a reasonable fee, via BITNET, INTERNET, PRODIGY and COMPUSERV. It may also be accessed through the European network EARN. For those who do not have access to any of these networks, NAPRALERT can provide off-line searches at competitive rates. The database is also available through Scientific and Technical Information Network (STN).

Fees: The NAPRALERT database is available on a scheduled fee basis to scientists, industrial firms, government agencies and to academic institutions. Requests should be made by completing the NAPRALERT ORDER FORM. A standard fee is applicable to ethnomedical, experimental biological activity and/or chemical constituent profiles, whether for one species, genus or family of organism. Other types of requests may require special programming and cost estimates are available on request.

Address: Department of Medicinal Chemistry and Pharmacognosy, College of Pharmacy of the University of Illinois at Chicago, 833 South Wood Street (M/C 877), Chicago, IL 60612, U.S.A. (Tel.: +1 / 312 / 996-2246, Fax: +1 / 312 / 996-7107, e-mail: Quinn@pcog.pmmp.uic.edu).

Contact through STN:

Europe: Scientific and Technical Information Network (STN), c/o FIZ (Fachinformationszentrum) Karlsruhe, Gelände des Forschungszentrums, 76344 Eggenstein-Leopoldshafen, Germany. Tel.: (+49) 7247 / 808-555, Fax: (+49) 7247 / 808-259.

Japan: STN International, c/o The Japan Information Centre of Science and Technology (JICST), 5-2, Nagatacho 2-chrome, Chiyoda-ku, Tokyo 100 Japan (Tel.: +81 / 3 / 3581-6448).

Pharmel

The Pharmel database is the result of one of the various projects of the *Agence de Coopération Culturelle et Technique* (ACCT). This agency is an intergovernmental francophone organization founded in 1970 that supports activities in technical cooperation, economic development, culture and education. In 1986, the ACCT entrusted the Département de Botanique systématique et de Phytosociologie, Université Libre de Bruxelles with the establishment and maintenance of the Pharmel database that would record information on traditional remedies in the different ACCT Member States.

Objective of the database is to conserve indigenous knowledge and to incorporate the traditional knowledge on medicinal plants in health systems of developing countries. More than 4000 plants used as traditional remedies are recorded, mainly from Central and Western Africa. The Pharmel database is planned to establish a network of local independant databases. The last update of the database was made in 1994. The database is held in French language, but an English version is established soon.

Contact address:

Professeur Jean Lejoly
Département de Botanique systématique et de Phytosociologie
Université Libre de Bruxelles
28, avenue Paul Héger

B-1050 Bruxelles
Belgium
Tel.: (+32) 2 / 6502126
Fax: (+32) 2 / 6502135

SEPASAL (Survey of Economic Plants for Arid and Semi-Arid Lands)

SEPASAL is a database on useful plants of drylands and is maintained by the Centre for Economic Botany at Royal Botanic Gardens, Kew. The database, founded in 1981, contains information on more than 6.000 useful dryland species, excluding major crops.

Data fields available include: sientific name, plant family, vernacular and trade name, plant description, geographical distribution, conservation status, life cycle and regeneration, uses of plants, use-related properties and chemical analysis, ecological data, physiology, cultivation details and seed sources. Distribution maps and colour images are provided as additional illustrations.

The value of the database depends on feedback from its users. Therefore, SEPASAL asks for further information on species of potential value in arid and semi-arid regions (short questionnaire available from address below).

Access to SEPASAL information is free for NGOs involved in development work. Charges are made to commercial enquirers. As methods of data dissemination, the possibilities of releasing CD-Rom versions of SEPASAL or Run-Time Versions of the software are being examined.

Two other databases are maintained by the Centre for Economic Botany. The *Economic Botany Bibliography Database* currently contains citations to more than 150,000 references dealing with plants of economic value. The *Contact's Database* has records of over 1000 organisations and projects mostly concerned with drylands.

For enquiries contact:

SEPASAL, Centre for Economic Botany
Royal Botanic Gardens, Kew
Richmond, Surrey TW9 3AE
U.K.
(manager: Mr. Frances Cook)
Tel.: (+44) 181 / 332-5772, - 5704
Fax: (+44) 181 / 332-5278
e-mail: sepasal@rbgkew.org.uk

Threatened Plants Database at World Conservation Monitoring Centre

Through its *Threatened Plants Database*, the World Conservation Monitoring Centre (WCMC), formerly operating as the IUCN Conservation Monitoring Centre, gathers, analyzes, and provides information on these plants, the only organization to do so on a global scale. This information is widely disseminated so that it may be used to make informed land- and species-management decisions.

This information resides in three forms:

- computerised databases: currently, WCMC holds taxonomic, distribution, and conservation information on more than 95,000 species of plants - over 1/3 of all described higher plants;
- manual files: approximately 20 m of box files and 40 file cabinet drawers containing published and unpublished reports, surveys, taxonomic descriptions, and correspondence; and
- cards: 68,000 cards track information about a plant's name, synonymy, distribution, conservation status, changes in status over time, and the data sources for the often conflicting information.

Since the late 1960s, WCMC has gathered two related plant taxon based data sets: all single-country endemics (those plants found growing naturally in only one country), no matter what their conservation status; and all other plants of conservation concern at the national level, no matter what their level of endemism. Many other datasets are maintained or are being developed, notably the development of a world tree list, and crosslinkages to record information from protected area inventories and legislation on the protection provided to named taxa.

Plant information comes to WCMC from a variety of sources and in a variety of formats. Published and unpublished reports, Red Data Books, and Red Data Lists are scanned and the relevant information entered into the databases. Correspondence with several thousand contacts worldwide, particularly members of IUCN's Species Survival Groups, also supplies important information. Increasingly, data comes already computerised, often using internationally agreed transfer protocols, enabling this data to be incorporated electronically. Likewise, plant information is output either on paper or electronically in a variety of forms - geographically or taxonomically structured conservation listings, bibliographies, statistical tables, status summaries, etc.

Although the *Threatened Plants Database* is not specifically for medicinal plants, there is a field in which species which are known to have a medicinal value are marked and so it should be possible to generate lists from these.

Address: World Conservation Monitoring Centre, 219 Huntingdon Road, Cambridge CB3 0DL, United Kingdom. Tel.: (+44) 1223 / 277-314, Fax: (+44) 1223 / 277-136.

Directory of Specialists

International Directory of Specialists in Herbs, Spices, and Medicinal Plants

The *International Directory of Specialists in Herbs, Spices, and Medicinal Plants* provides the addresses, phone and fax numbers, professional specialities, and associated plant material for individuals from 86 countries. The list covers professionals in botany, business, horticulture, medicine, pharmacology, processors, regulators, and others with an interest in aromatic and medicinal plants. Besides inclusion under a home country, each specialist is indexed alphabetically for easy reference.

The list of specialists was compiled from personal contacts of the editor. Individuals interested in some scientific, medical or business aspect of aromatic and medically useful plant species were located through the use of mailing lists, referrals, and literature references.

The second edition of this directory was published in 1994 and it is intended to update it.

Copies of the directory may be obtained at US-$ 35.00 (plus postage) from: Lyle E. Craker, The Herb, Spice, and Medicinal Plant Digest, Department of Soil Science, Stockbridge Hall, University of Massachusetts, Amherst, MA 01003, U.S.A.

Awards

The Richard Evans Schultes Award

To increase the visibility of the contributions of ethnobotany, and to foster and give due recognition to those who further the field, *The Healing Forest Conservancy* presents an annual award to a scientist, practitioner, or organization that has made an outstanding contribution to ethnobotany or to indigenous peoples issues related to ethnobotany. The award honours the name of *Richard Evans Schultes*, widely recognized as one of the most distinguished figures in the field. *Schultes* received the Annual Gold Medal of the World Wildlife Fund (today's World Wide Fund for Nature) from the organization's then-president, Prince Philip of the United Kingdom, the Tyler Prize for Environmental Achievement and the Linnean Gold Medal. *Schultes* has published among numerous papers in scientific journals „The Healing Forest" (1990), together with *Robert Raffauf.* The Healing Forest Conservancy is named after this book.

The International Nominating Committee for the award is chaired by Michael J. Balick, Director of the New York Botanical Garden's Institute of Economic Botany. The awards have been presented during meetings of the Society for Economic Botany, which was founded in 1959 as an international scientific organization to further ethnobotanical research and to disseminate results through meetings and publications.

To date, there have been three recipients of the Schultes Award. The late *Calvin R. Sperling*, of the National Germplasm Resources Laboratory at the US Department of Agriculture, was recognized in 1993 for his comprehensive work as a field ethnobotanist in the preservation of genetic resources and the ethnobotany of economic plants. The 1994 Schultes Award was presented to Professor *Hernando Garcia Barriga* of the Universidad de Colombia for the numerous students from the tropics that he trained and for his three-volume series „Flora Medicinal de Colombia". The Schultes Award for 1995 was presented to *Janis B. Alcon*, Director for Asia and the Pacific of the Biodiversity Support Program at the World Wildlife Fund in Washington, DC. The award recognizes her outstanding contribution in strengthening indigenous peoples' participation in community-based conservation of biological diversity.

Each Schultes Award has featured a US-$ 5000 cash prize donated by *Shaman Pharmaceuticals*, Inc. and *The Leland Fikes Foundation*, Inc. The Foundation, located in Dallas, supports local biomedical research and has a general interest in biodiversity as a part of the broad field of medicine. The Healing Forest Conservancy, which sponsors the

Schultes Award, was founded by Shaman Pharmaceuticals, Inc., a natural products company in South San Francisco, California, focussed on the discovery and development of pharmaceuticals through ethnobotany. The Conservancy, a non-profit foundation, is dedicated to the conservation of tropical forests, particularly medicinal plants and their sustainable use for human health. The focus of the Conservancy is to deliver compensation programmes that strengthen the integrity of traditional cultures to native communities that have participated in Shaman's drug discovery process.

The Richard Evans Schultes Award seeks a balance in geographic location, gender and field of study for recipients. Nominations of indigenous people active in this area are especially welcome.

Further information, including the deadine for nominations, is available from: Katy Moran, Executive Director, The Healing Forest Conservancy, 3521 S Street, N.W., Washington, D.C. 20007, U.S.A. Fax : (+1) 202 / 333-3438.

Egon Stahl Award

On the occasion of his 60th birthday, Professor Dr. Dr. h.c. mult. Egon Stahl donated a medal, a certificate and a monetary prize to recognize and promote young scientists working in the field of Pharmacognosy (Pharmaceutical Biology) and Analytical Phytochemistry.

As a rule, the silver medal and an award of DM 4000 (at present) is awarded to scientists up to the age of about forty who have published outstanding scientific work during the years after their graduation.

The bronze medal and an award of DM 3000 (at present) will be given to young scholars up to the age of about thirty whose theses are of outstanding quality.

Normally, the prize for outstanding scientific work will be awarded annually by the President or the Vice President of the Society for Medicinal Plant Research, at a special ceremony held as a part of the congress of that society.

Members of the Society for Medicinal Plant Research may submit nominations for candidates, together with supporting data, to the President of the Society.

Information on the deadlines for nominations is available from:

Society for Medicinal Plant Research, The President, Prof. Dr. Gerhard Franz, University of Regensburg, Faculty of Chemistry and Pharmacy, Universitätsstr. 31, 93053 Regensburg, Germany. Tel.: (+49) 941 / 943-4760, Fax: (+49) 941 / 943-4762, e-mail: Gerhard.Franz@chemie.uni-regensburg.de.

Index
Groups listed in alphabetic order

Country Index